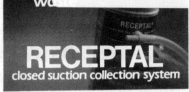

Ase
colle
and d
of me
suc
wa

RECEPTAL®
closed suction collection system

The Receptal® system for the collection of medical suction waste differs from other systems by incorporating a unique sealed liner.

The suction waste is collected in a tough PVC liner, which is sealed to its own lid. This enables the collection and disposal of the suction waste without the contents coming into contact with the outside air.

The liner and contents can then simply be incinerated.

The Receptal® system may be used for the aseptic collection and disposal of all medical suction waste. Its closed system will afford

greater protection for patients against cross contamination especially with staphylococcal infections, in open bowel surgery, tuberculosis and Australia antigen cases – the latter two being of special importance to the health of hospital staff.

For further details please contact:—

Clinical Products Division
Abbott Laboratories Limited, Queenborough, Kent ME11 5EL
Telephone: Sheerness (0795) 663371

RECEPTAL®–
THE DIFFERENCE IS IN THE LINER

"GET WELL SOON. THAT'S AN ORDER".

Seriously though, no-one joins the QA's to play at soldiers.

We are, first and foremost, nurses. Caring not only for the military, but their wives and families, and some civilian cases.

Our nursing experience ranges from midwifery at Aldershot to tropical illnesses in Hong Kong. We also train girls to become RGN's.

If you'd like to find out more about life in the QA's, drop us a line and we'll send you our full brochure.

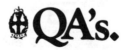 **QA's.**

Baillière's Ward Information

Douglas Middleton

SRN, RNT, DipEd(Lond)
Nurse Tutor
Charles Frears School of Nursing,
Leicester

Fourteenth Edition

Baillière Tindall
London Philadelphia Toronto

Published by Baillière Tindall
1 St Anne's Road, Eastbourne
East Sussex BN21 3UN

First published 1933 as *The Nurse's Pharmacopoeia*
  by Dr H. L. Heimann and Dora Wilson
Seventh edition 1953 as *Pocket Book of Ward Information*
  by Marjorie Houghton
Thirteenth edition 1980
Fourteenth edition 1984

Typeset by Photo-Graphics, Honiton, Devon
Printed and bound in Great Britain by
William Clowes Limited, Beccles and London

British Library Cataloguing in Publication Data

Baillière's ward information.—14th ed.
  1. Nursing
  I. Middleton, Douglas
  610.73   RT41

ISBN 0–7020–1032–4

Preface

During the revision of this useful pocket-sized book for its 14th edition I have kept in mind the assiduous work of the previous authors, Marjorie Houghton and L. Ann Jee. In keeping with the tradition they have set, the book remains full of facts, figures, definitions and basic procedures fundamental to the practice of nursing. The text can be used either as a quick reference or 'aide memoire' while actually on duty or as a basic study guide or companion to larger and more comprehensive nursing texts.

The developments in the nursing profession since the 13th edition include the re-organization of the structure of the National Health Service and the establishment of the United Kingdom Central Council for Nurses, which replaces the former General Nursing Councils. This latter change brings together under one organization all the previously separate trainings offered to general and specialist groups of nurses. A great deal of emphasis is now placed on the need for continuous education throughout a nursing career in addition to the statutory training schemes, which will undoubtedly be reviewed in the coming months and years.

Concurrent with these changes has been the continuing development of a philosophy of care as outlined in 'The Nursing Process' which uses a problem solving approach. The goal is to attempt to meet the individual needs of each sick person. However, to attain this the nurse in training needs a sound core of basic but accurate information accessible in a quick and ready manner. The author hopes this small text will meet this need.

During the review of this book I received help and advice from many colleagues, both in the District School of Nursing and in the acute hospitals of the Leicester District Health Authority, for which I am most grateful.

Douglas Middleton   *August 1983*

Contents

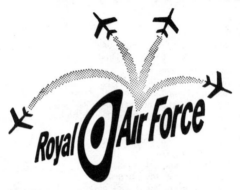

1
Professional Nursing

Elementary to the foundation of professionalism in nursing is an appreciation of those features common to all nurses throughout the world. These are listed by the International Council of Nurses as being:

1. To provide care in a suitable environment which protects the values, customs and spiritual beliefs of the patient.
2. To value, respect and hold in confidence privileged information, and exercise judgement concerning with whom such information is shared.
3. To achieve skilled practice and be personally responsible for safe competence in the giving of care.
4. To achieve the highest realistic standard of competence in the giving of care.
5. To maintain standards of personal conduct which reflect credit on the individual nurse and the nursing profession.
6. To share the responsibility of supporting measures which meet the health needs of the public.
7. To take appropriate action to safeguard the individual patient when their care is endangered by a colleague or other person.
8. To implement desirable standards of nursing care and be personally responsible for developing a core of knowledge.
9. To participate in promoting equitable social and economical working conditions for all nurses.

Extrapolated from these ideals are several distinctive elements which the nurse is expected to continually develop in order to attain professionalism. The clinical, coordinating, counselling and research aspects of any branch of nursing are based on sound and factual knowledge. Such knowledge can only be obtained from a wide study of the many available resources in the nursing library and an acceptance of personal responsibility to achieve understanding. The nurse must go beyond the clinical experience gained from day to day and seek out its link with theoretical concepts. The ultimate objective of both knowledge and skill is that nursing practice is not only seen to be, but is actually, safe. Safety in practice requires the nurse to be conscientious, not only in recording measurements but in all nursing procedures, including the courteous and kind attitudes expected of the nurse towards patients and their relatives, peers and senior colleagues.

2
Notes on Ward Administration

Upon entering nurse training, the nurse is best advised to look for those similarities which exist between the many types of ward in which he or she will work.

Policy and Procedures

On every ward the nurse should find two important files. The first of these will refer to hospital policy. Many of the policies outlined give guidelines in everyday routine matters and the procedure for emergencies such as fire. The policies can be regarded as rules, which are very necessary if any institution such as a hospital is to run effectively and efficiently. The second file will deal with nursing procedures. While such procedures will be demonstrated and the nurse can expect to be supervised, the files are always there for those unexpected occasions when the nurse is called upon to carry out an unusual procedure. The nurse may also find on each ward a list of learning objectives. This will guide nurses in training as to what they are expected to learn when allocated to a particular ward.

Ward Accidents

Every member of the nursing staff has a duty to ensure that nursing practice is conducted in a safe environment. The risk of accidents to patients or staff must be minimized by careful examination of each nursing situation. Spillage on floors, faulty electrical equipment, loose carpeting and badly-sited furniture are all matters that can be dealt with quickly and effectively. However, accidents do occur despite the best precautions and the nurse must know the local policy with regard to accidents to patients, visitors or staff. Generally, the patient is reassured and returned to bed. The medical officer should examine the patient and will order investigations or treatment. The nursing staff must complete an accident form and where possible this should be countersigned by a witness to the accident. The doctor may also be asked to sign the form. The unit nursing officer is notified and should retain the accident form for record purposes. All accidents occurring in the ward should be investigated by the nursing staff. Any significant change in ward procedure which would help to prevent similar accidents in the future should be reported to the unit nursing officer for agreement and approval.

Written Consent

Many routine treatments are carried out with the patient's verbal or implied consent. However, written consent is required for the administration of anaesthesia. The legal age for written consent is 16 years. Many surgeons prefer the joint signatures of husband and wife for many gynaecological or obstetric procedures. In cases of abortion the parents' written consent may also be asked for even though the patient is over 16 years of age. In the case of children, the parent or legal guardian is asked to sign the consent form. For surgery, the houseman is normally responsible for explaining the reasons for surgery and witnessing the patient's signature.

Diet

The nurse will soon notice that diet plays an important part in the treatment plan of many patients. The nutritional needs of the patient are the joint responsibility of the dietician and the nursing staff. It is important to know not only which patients are on special diets but also those patients who are temporarily fasting because of surgery or investigations. It is equally important to appreciate that the patient's religion may involve some dietary restriction.

The introduction of the plated meal service has reduced the amount of work for the nurse but it in no way absolves the nurse of the responsibility for ensuring that the correct diet is given to the right patient and that helpless patients are kept in good nutritional balance by expert feeding techniques and good observation.

Supplies

Normally the type and location of equipment follows a standard pattern throughout the hospital. It is worthwhile getting to know the method of supply, handling and disposal of equipment. Many hospital departments maintain full stock by a daily or weekly replenishing system, e.g. the pharmacy, linen room and sterile supplies department.

It is important for the nurse to learn to distinguish disposable and non-disposable items as soon as possible. For example, some surgical instruments are disposable after several episodes of being sterilised whereas stainless steel items are continuously recycled. Breakages and/or faulty equipment should always be reported to senior staff who will advise on replacement or repair. Only after taking advice should damaged equipment be thrown away.

Admission

The admission of patients to hospital requires two very important principles to be observed.

Firstly, the hospital cannot accept total responsibility for a patient's property. The patient should be encouraged to return unnecessary items to his or her home with a relative and the nurse should list all items the patient wishes to retain in hospital; this is even more important when admitting an unconscious patient. Such a list should preferably be witnessed by another nurse. Large sums of money, for which the patient will be given a receipt, can be secured in the hospital safe. For very short periods only, a ward sister/charge nurse can lock away valuables, such as watches, in his or her office cupboard.

Secondly, every patient admitted to hospital should have an identity band attached to his/her wrist. The information on the band will include the patient's name, age, ward and hospital number. The correct identification of patients in busy acute hospitals cannot be emphasized enough.

Records

Nursing records are standard throughout a hospital. The charting of nursing observations must be accurate and legible and comply with the frequency requested by the doctor. Such records are used extensively to monitor the patient's progress and may also determine changes in treatment. Nursing reports, usually in Kardex form, should be available to all nursing staff, and are especially important when shift work patterns operate.

The patient's notes are confidential and should be treated as privileged information; they must never leave the ward without the ward sister's/charge nurse's knowledge. All nursing reports will be retained in the patient's file until it is destroyed; this time varies with each authority.

Nurses should never offer or give information to the Press about those patients in their care.

Visiting Times

Hospital visiting times vary from ward to ward. In a children's ward free visiting is the normal pattern, in order to help maintain the normal child–parent relationship. Free visiting is also allowed for the very seriously ill patient, with overnight accommodation and catering facilities being offered to the relatives if required.

Visiting times are very important to the patient but can be very tiring; discretion can be used by the nurse to end a visit.

Relatives seeking an interview with medical staff should be referred to the senior nurse on duty who will arrange an interview with the doctor.

Chaplains

Every hospital offers a chaplaincy service to patients and staff alike. The appointed chaplains visit the wards on a regular basis and normally respond to requests to console bereaved relatives. Those patients who are Hindu, Moslem, Jewish or Catholic should have their wishes respected regarding dietary restrictions and also their customs about the last rites. It is also worth noting that children's wards have a special way of dealing with baptism and with the deceased child.

Wills

Regardless of where the nurse works, under no circumstances should he or she sign a will; if necessary this will be done by the hospital secretarial staff.

Nursing Methods

The day-to-day administration of the ward and the nursing method employed is the responsibility of the ward sister/charge nurse. As the training nurse moves from one allocation to the next he or she may be apprehensive about working effectively within differing styles of nursing method. Such nursing style depends on the size of the ward, the type of patient and the training needs of nursing staff.

Formerly the most common method of working was 'task allocation', where each nurse would be given a series of tasks, not necessarily related to direct nursing care, to do within his or her span of duty. This style of working is still valid in departmental work, e.g. outpatients, theatre and clinics, and may be used in conjunction with the 'nursing process' for smooth ward administration.

'Patient allocation' requires a nurse to care for an individual patient or group of patients, usually working on his or her own. This method is not popular with junior nurses, who feel insecure without the support of senior colleagues. For experienced nurses who have been given good in-service training working with critically ill patients, this method of working is most rewarding.

On the main wards, team nursing is the most obvious choice. In this system the ward staff are grouped into teams, usually led by a staff nurse who coordinates the work of his or her team in the care of a group of patients. One major drawback is that if the team is to work consistently and cohesively it needs to have at its core permanent members of staff who can build up a sense of belonging and purpose. Part time staff may have difficulty in fitting into a pattern of team nursing.

The 'nursing process' is the most recent innovation in nursing style and is designed to provide total nursing care.

The nursing process (Figure 1) The philosophy of this nursing method utilises four skills which the nurse

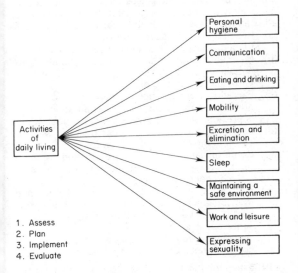

Figure 1. The nursing process

should be constantly developing during his/her training period. These skills are:

1. Interviewing a patient to assess their individual needs.
2. Planning the care to meet the assessed needs.
3. Implementing the devised plan of care.
4. Evaluating the care plan at frequent intervals, introducing changes as and when required.

1. *Interviewing the patient.* The initial interview should always be based upon the 'activities of daily living', in order to assess whether these activities are impeded because of the illness. Basic activities which the healthy adult takes for granted, but which may be affected by illness, include the following:

(a) Respiration. This takes priority over all other body functions, especially if the airway is threatened.
(b) Maintaining nutrition. This includes the ability to handle crockery and cutlery, and cope with a particular prescribed diet.
(c) Excretion from the bowel, bladder or skin. The nurse not only assesses whether an abnormality is present, but also how the patient copes with it.
(d) Locomotor skills. This includes posture, walking and fine movements of the hands.
(e) Communication. This may be affected by deafness, speech defects, partial or total blindness, or reduced consciousness.
(f) Expressing individuality, personal identity and individual sexuality. An altered body image may lead to considerable emotional distress.
(g) A normal sleep pattern.
(h) Work and leisure. Illness may affect social or work commitments, or the home environment.

The aim of the interview is to establish how the patient as an individual sees his/her own problems rather than imposing an assumed generalization obtained from the nurse's experience. Standard assessment forms are usually available on most training wards for use during the initial interview.

In addition to obtaining essential basic information, the nurse should consider the style and duration of the first interview. It should be informal, with the nurse sitting at the bedside so that eye to eye contact with the patient is possible. The interview should not exceed 15 minutes at any one time; too long an interview may cause anxiety. The tone of the interview should be that of 'between equals'. Dominating the situation or being too submissive may prevent the collection of vital information. A careful study of the interview form will help the nurse ask some introductory questions without constantly referring to a piece of paper and will also help maintain eye to eye contact. A second interview may be necessary to elucidate any obscure points, especially when the nurse is not satisfied with the fine detail or the clarity and consistency of answers given. It is sometimes necessary to interview the relatives if the patient is uncooperative or unconscious.

The information obtained will be used to formulate a plan of care tailored to meet the individual's needs while in hospital.

2. *Planning the care.* The nursing plan should be based on the *patient's* needs, which are assessed during the initial interview. The plan should also take into account the prescribed medical regimen. Planning the care consists of:
(a) Stating the goal or aim to be achieved.
(b) Identifying the clinical care required to achieve the stated goal.
(c) Stating the expected outcome of any care given.

A successful plan would take into account a 24 hour period of time and thus meet all the patient's needs within one day.

3.   *Implementing the care.*   This phase of the nursing process covers the clinical and managerial skills needed to meet the plan of care. A great deal of it is the 'doing' of procedures within the agreed ward or hospital policy guidelines. Whilst implementing the care, the ability to plan, to give skilled attention and to work out the patient's priorities are tested.

4.   *Evaluating the care.*   Experience has shown that this is one of the most difficult concepts for the nurse in training to grasp. When a plan is evaluated, the degree of success or failure of care is expressed in objective terms and not as an opinion or assumption. Routine observations such as temperature, pulse, blood pressure, weight, urinalysis and respiration rate are all easily expressed in objective terms. The difficulty arises when the nurse is asked to evaluate progress in factors such as locomotor ability or wound healing. However, these can be accurately measured using a combination of theoretical knowledge and observational skills.

If a plan of care is not successful, the nursing team must go back and look at it carefully to discover why, and change it so that the original goal or aim is finally achieved.

From experience it is being found that this method is most successful with those patients requiring long-term care either in hospital or in the community. It is a very valuable method from which nurses can develop a deep awareness of total nursing care in a team situation.

3
Ward Emergencies and Related Procedures

Immediate action to be taken in some common emergencies is summarized in Table I on page 22.

The nurse may be involved in an emergency situation in which an important decision must be taken quickly. Each hospital lays down its own policy about the responsibilities that an individual nurse may assume; it is very important that the nurse becomes acquainted with hospital policy, especially on emergencies, at the earliest opportunity. Unless it is absolutely unavoidable the nurse must seek advice from a doctor or senior member of nursing staff. If this is impossible, the nurse should ask another nurse to witness his/her actions. In any case the nurse must always report to a senior colleague at the earliest opportunity any decision taken on his/her own initiative.

Whatever the emergency, the ability to think clearly and remain calm is a valuable asset; shouting and confusion not only frighten patients but may upset other members of the ward team.

Collapse

If a patient should collapse, from whatever cause, the immediate principles to follow are:

- Check that the patient's airway is clear.

- Summon help from colleagues.

- Ensure that the resuscitation trolley is available and ready for use.

- Treat for shock. (If giving oxygen, see Oxygen Therapy, p. 33.)

At the first appropriate moment reassure the patient and those in the vicinity. The nurse should also remember the collapsed patient may still hear what is being said.

Cardiac Arrest

The sudden, unexpected and total failure of the heart to pump blood around the body is known as cardiac arrest. Common causes are post-operative shock, myocardial infarction and coronary thrombosis (common in the first 24 hours following the initial attack), electrocution, and drug overdose. The brain is the organ most sensitive to lack of oxygen. Brain cells at normal body temperature will die if the circulation is not restored within 3–4 minutes. The obvious signs that a patient has suffered a cardiac arrest are:

- Sudden collapse and unconsciousness.
- Gasping or absent respiration.
- Greyish cyanosis with pallor developing later.
- Dilated pupils.
- Twitching and a brief major fit in some cases.
- Absent radial and femoral pulses.

The cardiac arrest team must be alerted without delay.

Cardiac Resuscitation

- **Summon help immediately** by dialling the emergency telephone number, while a second nurse remains with the patient.
- **Place the patient on a hard surface** e.g. Fracture boards placed beneath the mattress.
- **Clear the airway of any foreign material**, especially dentures.

- **Elevate the lower limbs** to aid the return of venous blood.
- **Give a sharp blow to the lower sternum;** this may restart the heart.
- If it does not, **begin external cardiac massage:**
  —Place one hand flat on the lower sternum.
  —Place the heel of the other hand over it.
  —With the arms straight, press downwards over the lower end of the sternum. A rhythmic swinging forward movement of the shoulders depresses the sternum by about 4 cm. This squeezes the heart against the vertebral column.
  —Repeat this movement about 60 times per minute.
- **Mouth-to-mouth respiration** is also begun immediately (see p. 17). *One* lung inflation should alternate with *six* chest compressions.
- If only one nurse is present, *three* lung inflations should alternate with *fifteen* chest compressions.
- While cardiac massage and mouth-to-mouth respiration are continued:
  —Fetch the **resuscitation trolley.**
  —Screen off the area.
  —Remove furniture and other obstacles to make room for the cardiac arrest team.
- Mouth-to-mouth resuscitation is replaced by **a Brook airway with an Ambu bag attached** as soon as this is available.
- **On arrival of the cardiac arrest team** the respiratory function is taken over by the anaesthetist, who will pass an endotracheal tube and attach the Ambu bag to continue inflating the chest.
- A second doctor will establish **an intravenous infusion,** usually of sodium bicarbonate 8.4%, and will also use this route to administer drugs **which the nurse will draw up in readiness.**
- External cardiac massage is continued throughout.

- **Limb or chest electrodes attached to a cardiac monitor** may be used to give continuous monitoring of the heart beat.
- **The defibrillating machine** may be used to pass an electrical current through the chest wall to the heart to establish the heart beat or correct an arrhythmia. During defibrillation external cardiac massage is stopped for a few seconds.
- The doctor will continually check the femoral pulse and the heart's rhythm on the cardiac monitor to determine when external massage should stop.

It is usual for those who have been successfully resuscitated to be transferred to the intensive care unit for further treatment. Following this emergency it is important to contact and inform the next of kin.

It is necessary for the nurse to appreciate that other patients witnessing any part of this procedure are very alarmed and distressed. During the procedure those nurses who are not immediately involved can reassure the other patients and continue the normal work pattern.

N.B. To perform cardiac massage in infants both thumbs are applied over the midline of the sternum and light compression (12 mm) is applied at the rate of 100–120 per minute.

Asphyxia

When breathing stops through interference with the normal levels of oxygen and carbon dioxide in the body, this may be due to obstruction of the airway, paralysis of the respiratory muscles caused by drugs, gases, or disease, collapse of lung tissue, or replacement of air content by fluid, e.g. drowning or inhaled vomit. If the airway is obstructed and the patient can stand, a simple method of removing the obstruction is:

- Stand behind the patient.
- Bring your arms forward around in front of the patient.
- Clench one hand into a fist.
- Use the other hand to bring the fist sharply into the central upper abdomen just below the diaphragm, applying an upper abdominal thrust.
- Such a blow should eject the obstruction from the pharynx into the mouth.

For other cases of asphyxia artificial ventilation is required. Many methods are available, some suitable for emergency situations and for short periods only, others for longer periods.

Artificial Airways

In most hospitals a Brook airway is readily available. This is similar to the airway used in anaesthetized patients, but it contains a seal to cover the patient's mouth and a one-way valve. This is preferable to direct mouth-to-mouth artificial respiration, particularly if the patient has a chest infection. Many hospitals provide a simple type of self-inflating bag, e.g. an Ambu bag which can be attached to the Brook airway. This can be used in emergencies until medical help arrives.

Mouth-to-Mouth and Mouth-to-Nose Artificial Respiration

- Lie the patient on his/her back with the nurse standing level with the patient's head at the bedside, or kneeling if the patient is on the floor.

- Quickly clear the mouth and throat of any foreign material, particularly dentures.
- With one hand on the patient's forehead and the other under the neck, tilt the patient's head as far back as possible. This position is maintained throughout the procedure.
- Form a wide seal over the patient's mouth with your lips, pressing your cheek against the patient's nose to seal the nasal passages. The nostrils may be pinched together.
- Blow air into the mouth until the patient's chest rises. The patient is allowed to breath out spontaneously.
- The first ten breaths are given rapidly, and then the rate should be between 12 and 15 breaths per minute.
- Alternatively, the mouth may be sealed, and air blown into the nose; it is said there is less likelihood of blowing air into the stomach by this method.

N.B. In infants and babies the lips should cover both the patient's mouth and nose. The nurse must breathe gently and not too deeply if damage to the delicate lung tissue is to be avoided.

Pulmonary Embolism

Pulmonary embolism occurs when a blood clot (usually from a deep vein thrombosis) becomes detached, travels in the venous circulation, and blocks a blood vessel in the lungs. The embolism may alternatively be due to fat, released from a broken bone, or to air accidentally introduced into the venous circulation during intravenous therapy. Blood clots usually originate from the pelvic or deep calf veins. Pulmonary embolism may follow surgery, particularly that undertaken in the pelvic area, may be associated with congestive heart failure, or may be a consequence of prolonged bedrest.

The severity of symptoms produced depends on the size of the clot. It may vary from slight chest pain, breathlessness and cyanosis to a sudden fatal collapse.

If pulmonary embolism is suspected the nurse should:

- Assist the patient into a position which will make respiration easier and more comfortable.
- **Administer oxygen quickly.** The venti-mask must be used for patients with respiratory disease, cor pulmonale or congestive cardiac failure.
- **Summon the doctor** so that appropriate therapy may be started as soon as possible.
- **Reassure the patient** as he/she will be very frightened and have a feeling of imminent catastrophe.

Sudden Haemorrhage

Haemorrhage, massive haematemesis or haemoptysis may follow an operation as a result of a ligature slipping from a main vessel. External bleeding is very obvious, but internal haemorrhage may be suspected from low blood pressure recordings and a rapid pulse or if the patient is restless for no apparent reason. Medical aid must be sought at once; any delay in replacing lost blood could prove fatal to the patient.

No patient suffering from haemorrhage should ever be left alone, and treatment for shock is essential (see below).

Treatment for Shock

Cardiac arrest, asphyxia, pulmonary embolism and sudden haemorrhage are all usually accompanied by severe shock, which needs to be treated as soon as breathing and heart beat have been restored.

Shock is defined simply as a decrease in the effective circulating blood volume or acute hypotension. The treatment will be of the cause, but a nurse can help by ensuring that the patient has a clear airway, is lying flat (in most cases), and is covered without being overheated. In severe shock the patient's veins may collapse quickly, making the administration of intravenous fluids more difficult. It is time-saving if the nurse can have the intravenous equipment ready for when the doctor arrives. Under no circumstances should oral fluids be given without the doctor's permission.

Blood pressure is lowered in cases of shock but it may also be lowered by the action of drugs given specifically by the anaesthetist during surgery. When a low blood volume persists after surgery, venous return is assisted by elevating the foot of the bed. Blood flow is more important than blood pressure in these particular cases but the nurse's observations are important and a systolic blood pressure recording below 60 mmHg must be reported to the doctor immediately.

Attempted Suicide

A patient may attempt to commit suicide in many ways. The observant nurse may well sense the patient's intention and so anticipate the action. Clear thinking, a calm manner, and a firm approach are of more value than stern or censorious behaviour towards a patient on the verge of suicidal action. A nurse who is alone should never attempt to restrain a patient who is violent or agitated, except to prevent him or her from harming other patients. Planned restraint with several assistants and the use of prescribed sedation may be necessary. Patients admitted after attempting suicide should be nursed in an open-plan ward with continuous observation. The patient with severe depression may be contemplating suicide, and the informed nurse taking an interest in such a patient can give invaluable psychological support and help to prevent this emergency.

All patients admitted after attempting suicide or making an attempt while in hospital should be referred for psychiatric opinion.

Fire Hazards

The nurse should quickly familiarize herself with the fire regulations which are prominently displayed throughout all hospitals. Fire doors should be kept shut at all times. In the event of fire they contain the smoke in the area affected. A knowledge of the location of the fire extinguishers on the ward, and how to use them, may prevent a small fire becoming an inferno. Ward kitchens should have a fire blanket available in case of fire from electric or gas ovens. Each bed should have a fire-proof evacuation sheet below the mattress; this is used to evacuate the bed-ridden patient from places where the patient's bed cannot be wheeled, e.g. fire escapes. Every ward has an emergency exit or fire escape, and these should never be blocked by laundry or furniture. Cigarette smoking is one of the principal causes of fires, and smoking should only be allowed in restricted areas and never on a ward.

Following the order to evacuate an area on fire, doors and windows should be closed and electrical appliances switched off if time permits. The main danger of fire is the resulting smoke, which causes suffocation; it is sometimes of more value to contain this by keeping doors closed than it is to contain the fire itself.

As an employee of the hospital the nurse should be familiar with the Health and Safety at Work Act 1979. All employers are required to organize annual lectures and demonstrations as part of in service training with regard to fire hazards which every hospital employee is required to attend.

Table I. Outline of action for some common emergencies

Emergency	Danger	Action
Asphyxia (see p.16)	Cardiac arrest, cerebral anoxia	1. Clear airway 2. Give artificial respiration 3. Treat for shock
Cardiac arrest (see p.14)	Brain death in 3–4 minutes unless circulation is restored	1. Clear airway 2. Lay patient on firm surface 3. Commence cardiac massage simultaneously with artificial respiration 4. Summon cardiac arrest team 5. Use any resuscitation equipment available

Emergency	Danger	Action
Pulmonary embolism (see p. 18)	Fatal collapse	1. Assist patient into comfortable position to aid respiration 2. Administer oxygen 3. Summon doctor 4. Reassure patient
Sudden haemorrhage (see p.19)	Circulatory collapse	1. Apply pressure directly or indirectly, if possible 2. Prepare for intravenous therapy 3. Administer oxygen 4. Elevate foot of bed 5. Prepare patient for theatre if indicated 6. Reassure patient 7. Prepare to give drugs i.v. or i.m.

N.B. In all cases treat for shock and follow hospital policy for dealing with emergencies.

4
Cardiac Monitors

Once attached to the patient a cardiac monitor gives a continuous visual or printed record of the heart's rhythm. This type of monitoring is frequently employed for patients suffering from recent heart attacks, after cardiac surgery or cardiac arrest, or to monitor the effect of implanted cardiac pacemakers.

The junior nurse is not expected to master the intricacies of the machine until proper training and instruction has been given, but all nurses should familiarize themselves with the essential controls and be able to appreciate whether a continuous tracing is showing a gross deviation. Cardiac monitors do not replace the other observations which the nurse must make; blood pressure, pulse rate, respiration, skin colour and pain are of equal importance and must also be reported upon at frequent intervals.

The monitoring equipment has two main cables. One leads from the main socket to the machine, the second goes from the machine to the patient and carries from three to five leads. Each lead carries a terminal at its tip. To these terminals are attached disposable electrodes which are applied to the patient's skin. When an electrocardiograph tracing is being taken the electrodes are flat metal discs applied to the ankles and wrists and held in place by rubber straps. For continuous cardiac monitoring, chest electrodes are used. The two most commonly used are the Dracard type, which requires to be changed daily, and the Optical type which can be left on the skin indefinitely. Both types must have electrode jelly applied to their adhesive backing before being applied to the patient's skin.

Once the equipment is prepared, the patient must be reassured as to the reason for monitoring the heart's rhythm. He/she can be told that all the machine does is to detect the electrical activity of the heart and that it is an excellent guide to the effectiveness of treatment that the patient is receiving. Before the electrodes are applied the chest wall may need to be shaved and the skin must be free of skin oils and as dry as possible. The position of the electrodes is decided by the doctor, but in an emergency these instructions can be followed:

When using a four-lead cable, apply the electrodes in the following positions
1. Third intercostal space to the right of the sternum.
2. Third intercostal space to the left of the sternum.
3. Sixth intercostal space to the right of the sternum.
4. Sixth intercostal space to the left of the sternum.
When using a three-lead cable, apply the electrodes diagonally from right to left across the anterior chest wall, moving from the third intercostal space on the right to the sixth intercostal space on the left.

When the machine is operational the controls are set by the doctor. The screen or oscilliscope must be facing away from the patient and the audible heart beat and alarm systems need not be used unless the patient is being left on his own for any length of time, which would be unusual since patients requiring monitoring are usually acutely ill. Should the tracing on the screen appear abnormal when the patient is alright, there is a fault in the cable, the leads or the electrodes which requires adjustment. Because the cables and leads are sometimes heavy and tend to get in the way, they should be pinned securely to the side of the mattress. Observations are best made by the same nurse over a span of duty; the minimal frequency of observation should be hourly and a minimum of six cardiac cycles should be observed.

The classical tracing of the heart's rhythm is shown in Figure 2. There can be normal variations to this classical pattern, but the patterns outlined in Figure 3 are examples of gross deviations which must be reported immediately because they indicate cardiac arrest requiring immediate resuscitation.

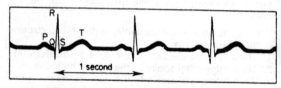

Figure 2.   The normal ECG trace. The P wave is the electrical conductivity of the sino-atrial node and the contraction of the atria. The QRS segment is the electrical conductivity resulting in ventricular contraction. The T segment is the electrical conductivity resulting from ventricular relaxation.

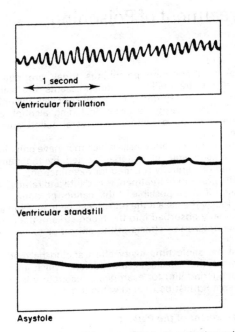

Figure 3. Abnormal ECG traces which indicate that immediate resuscitation is needed

5
Treatment of Poisoning

The most common poisonings today are due to hypnotics, tranquillizers, antidepressants and salicylates (such as aspirin). In many cases of self-poisoning a mixture of drugs is taken, including alcohol, and there may be a history of several failed suicide attempts.

All containers or utensils which may have contained the poison and all material ejected by the patient should be carefully retained for examination.

The first aim of treatment is to dilute and remove the poison if at all possible. If this cannot be done, as is obviously the case if the poison has been injected and is already absorbed into the blood stream, the aim is to neutralize the effects of the poison or to render it inactive.

At the same time every effort should be made to combat the effects of the poison, which may be endangering life; for example, if respiratory failure is present it must be treated without delay.

Assessment of the Patient

The patient is assessed on the degree of unconsciousness and the presence or absence of other medical complications such as shock or respiratory failure. Some patients who have become habituated to a drug (for example, epileptics taking phenobarbitone) are able to tolerate a much higher blood level of the drug before becoming unconscious or suffering ill effects than those who are not habituated. Adults suffering from acute salicylate poisoning rarely become rapidly unconscious; therefore, even drowsiness must be regarded as a dangerous sign. Children are more likely to become drowsy or unconscious. If there is any doubt about the amount of drug ingested, biochemical assessment must be undertaken without delay.

A successful outcome in roughly 95% of cases of poisoning depends on intensive nursing care of the unconscious patient. The remaining 5% of cases will require more specialized techniques of treatment such as forced diuresis or dialysis.

Respiratory Failure

Respiratory failure is liable to occur in poisoning due to barbiturates and other hypnotic drugs, carbon monoxide or cyanide. Maintenance of a clear airway is essential, the patient being nursed in the lateral position. Some doctors prefer the head to be lower than the feet, particularly where there is a risk of aspiration of vomit. Depending on the degree of unconsciousness, a cuffed endotracheal tube may be inserted. If the patient is cyanosed, oxgyen should be given. If there is any risk of carbon dioxide retention, a Venturi mask should be used (see p. 37). Artificial respiration may be necessary and if this is required for more than about 30 minutes a mechanical respirator will be needed, for example the Minuteman respirator (see p. 38). Occasionally it may be necessary to give 0.4–1.2 mg of naloxone (Narcan) intravenously to stimulate respiration temporarily whilst other equipment is being prepared. Tracheostomy is seldom necessary unless endotracheal intubation is needed for longer than 48 hours.

Shock

If elevation of the lower limbs is ineffective in raising the systolic blood pressure above 90 mmHg, other treatment should be instituted. It is thought that various mechanisms operate in cases of poisoning to produce a reduction in the venous return to the heart. One way to restore blood pressure is to give a vasoconstrictor drug, such as metaraminol intramuscularly 5 mg at 20 minute intervals. Intravenous fluids are not always desirable unless forced diuresis is the method of treatment.

Dilution of the Poison

In the majority of cases water is the most readily available fluid for dilution of a swallowed poison. The patient should be encouraged to drink as much as possible – four tumblers or more. Milk is also a suitable diluent, particularly in the case of corrosive or irritant poisons, since it has a demulcent action, protecting the mucous membrane and hindering absorption.

Removal of the Poison

In cases of salicylate poisoning, providing the swallow reflex is present, thorough *gastric lavage* (with plain warm water at 38°C) is the most effective method of treatment within four to twelve hours of ingestion of the poison. Where other corrosive poisons have been swallowed gastric lavage may be cautiously undertaken in selected cases; a doctor's advice should be sought.

In cases of petrol or paraffin poisoning 30 ml of liquid paraffin should be swallowed prior to the lavage. The patient is encouraged to swallow milk to which approximately 5 g of sodium bicarbonate has been added after the lavage. Castor oil, if it is easily available, can be added to the lavage water in cases of phenol poisoning; it dissolves the phenol, thereby delaying absorption.

With conscious children who have swallowed tablets the simplest and most effective method of removing the poison is to wrap them in a blanket, place them face down over the knees and irritate the pharynx, causing the child to vomit.

Where possible in the unconscious patient, intubation with a cuffed endotracheal tube should precede the lavage. Lavage is then easier and the patient's position not so important. Where intubation is not possible, the patient is best positioned face down, with his head lower than his body, to avoid the risk of fluid being inhaled. A wide-bore gastric tube should be slightly lubricated and passed through the mouth. About 300 ml of water is passed through the funnel before being syphoned back.

Emetics are not as efficient as gastric lavage but may be the quickest remedy available. The immediate use of emetics is contra-indicated in corrosive poisoning. The most effective emetic is 15 ml of syrup of ipecacuanha followed by 200 ml of water, repeated after twenty minutes if vomiting has not occurred. **N.B.** Do not use liquid extract of ipecacuanha which is much stronger.

A tablespoonful of salt or mustard mixed in a tumbler of warm water may be given to adults, but the use of salt and water is no longer recommended in the treatment of poisoning in children.

The following are examples of treatment that may be employed if simpler methods prove inadequate:

1. *Forced diuresis.* Used for ethyl and methyl alcohol, long-acting barbiturates, bromide, chloral hydrate, dichloralphenazone, lithium, salicylates, primidone.

2. *Peritoneal dialysis.* Used for amphetamines, boric

acid, antibiotics, sodium chlorate, paraldehyde.

3. *Haemodialysis.* Used for ethyl and methyl alcohol, aniline, long- and short-acting barbiturates, boric acid, bromide, carbon tetrachloride, chloral hydrate, dichloralphenazone, ethchlorvynol, fluoride, lead, lithium, Mandrax, salicylates, mushroom, paracetamol (in the four hours following ingestion), antibiotics.

Poisons Information Service

In the United Kingdom the Poisons Information Service give advice and information to general practitioners and hospitals on the treatment of specific poisons. It covers substances used in the home, agriculture, industry, and medicine. A comparable service is also available in Europe, Australia and the United States of America. The British telephone numbers are:

Belfast	0232 40503
Birmingham	021 554 3801
Cardiff	0222 569200
Dublin (Eire)	0001 745588
Edinburgh	031 229 2477
Leeds	0532 430715
	0532 432799
London	01 407 7600
Newcastle upon Tyne	0632 325131

(24 hour voluntary service)

6
Oxygen Therapy

Oxygen is administered in those conditions where the normal supply of oxygen to the tissues cannot be maintained. This may be due to respiratory difficulties, circulatory failure, or the inability of the red blood cells to combine with oxygen, as happens in carbon monoxide poisoning. Examples of common conditions in which oxygen therapy is either essential or beneficial are pneumonia, emphysema, cardiac and thoracic surgery, congestive cardiac failure and any condition producing severe shock.

Fire Precautions

Although oxygen itself does not burn, any material which burns in air will burn much more readily if the concentration of oxygen in the air is increased; therefore certain precautions are necessary. Patients and visitors should be warned not to smoke or light matches in the vicinity and notices should be placed to this effect. No electrical bells, lights or heating pads should be allowed inside an oxygen tent. Children should not be given mechanical toys which could cause a spark. Hair should not be vigorously combed. Patients should not wear nylon and must not be rubbed with oil or spirit while the tent is in operation. Should such rubbing be necessary the oxygen flow must be stopped for the duration of the treatment.

No oil or grease of any description must be used on the oxygen cylinder fittings. The head of the cylinder should be cleaned before attaching the regulator.

Cylinders and Fittings

For purposes of identification, oxygen and other medical gas cylinders are painted in distinctive colours and the name and/or symbol of the gas is stencilled on the cylinder. Table II gives the standard colours as issued by the British Standards Institute.

Table II.   Identification of gas cylinders

		Colour	
Gas	Symbol	Shoulder	Body
Oxygen	O_2	White	Black
Nitrous oxide	N_2O	Blue	Blue
Cyclopropane	C_2H_6	Orange	Orange
Ethylene	C_2H_4	Violet	Violet
Helium	He	Brown	Brown
Nitrogen	N_2	Black	Grey
Oxygen and carbon dioxide mixture	$O_2 + CO_2$	White and grey	Black
Oxygen and helium mixture	$O_2 + He$	White and brown	Black
Air	—	White and black	Grey

Oxygen is stored in cylinders at a pressure of approximately 13800 kPa (2000 lb/in^2). This pressure is regulated by the reducing valve of the head mount once it is attached (see Figure 4). It is important to open the valve slightly before attaching the head mount to allow the oxygen flow to blow away any grit or dust. Cylinders fittings should be attached outside the ward, away from the patients. Cylinders may also be fitted with nebulizers containing either water to humidify the oxygen or aerosol drugs.

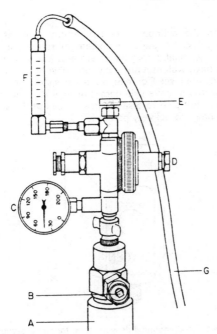

Figure 4. Oxygen cylinder fittings

A Cylinder (black body, white shoulder).
B Main valve. A spanner is used to open and close it.
C Pressure gauge. A zero reading, with the main valve open, means that the cylinder must be replaced immediately.
D Reducing valve (regulates pressure).
E Adjustment valve, used to obtain the prescribed rate of flow.
F Bobbin-type flow meter. Oxygen flow is measured in litres/minute.
G Tubing leading to disposable mask.

When the cylinder becomes empty it must be marked 'EMPTY' and a replacement requested immediately, usually from the pharmacy. Many hospital wards have wall-mounted oxygen delivery points for piped oxygen (see Figure 5), but there is still a need for such wards to have cylinders, not only as a standby measure but also to take to those areas of the ward which have no delivery points.

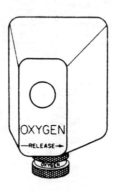

OXYGEN
←RELEASE→

Figure 5.   Wall-mounted delivery point for piped oxygen

Disposable Masks

Face masks are light in weight and durable. They cover both the nose and mouth. They may be rigid or flexible and soft. For maximum efficiency the mask must fit the patient's face closely but comfortably. Perspiration tends to accumulate on the patient's face and if this causes distress the mask can be lifted occasionally and the face quickly sponged. The rate of flow, ordered by the doctor, may vary between four and eight litres per minute.

Venti and Venturi masks have a rigid base with a flexible face area and are used for patients with chronic lung disease, which may be associated with chronic congestive cardiac failure. A rise in carbon dioxide concentration normally causes an increase in respiration. However, the respiratory centre in these patients has become conditioned to a higher concentration of carbon dioxide due to decreased oxygen intake. They therefore rely on a decreased oxygen concentration in the blood to stimulate respiration. A sudden large increase in the oxygen concentration could cause such patients to stop breathing. These masks are so constructed that the amount of oxygen the patient receives does not exceed 28% (in some cases 35%) at 4 litres per minute. This amount raises the level of oxygen in the blood sufficiently for the patient to benefit. Higher concentrations, such as those achieved by use of the oxygen tent or other face masks, could be fatal to these patients.

Many masks are perforated at the lower half of the face-piece which allows the patient to breathe a mixture of pure oxygen and air. This also allows some humidification of the pure oxygen to take place.

Nasal oxygen catheters have regained popularity. The catheter, shaped like a Y, is passed along the floor of the nose for 2.5 cm. This method of delivering oxygen increases the concentration that can be given, but there are associated discomforts for the patient. The oxygen tends to dry the mucous membranes, resulting in soreness. If necessary the nostrils may be cleaned with sodium bicarbonate solution and cocaine ointment applied to relieve the discomfort. Breathless patients tend to breathe through the mouth and would therefore benefit more from the use of a face

mask. The advantage of a nasal catheter is that the
mouth is left free for drinking, eating and, where
necessary, expectoration.

Mechanical Ventilators

There are now many types of mechanical ventilator
available for use when prolonged ventilation is necessary. The majority work on the principle of intermittent
positive pressure, and are attached to an endotracheal
tube for short periods, or a tracheostomy tube for
longer periods of mechanical ventilation.

These machines are constructed to pump air, oxygen or other gases rhythmically to and from the
patient's lungs. According to the various needs of the
patient, the machine can be regulated to control the
volume at inspiration and expiration. Some, known as
'breathing assisters', are triggered by the patient's
own breathing. The rate and pressure of breathing can
also be controlled, and the air can be humidified with
the aid of mechanical devices. These machines may at
first sight appear very complicated to the unpractised
nurse, but given the opportunity to observe the
machine in action, together with instructions regarding the function of the appropriate valves, the nurse
can soon become familiar with the aspects important
to the successful nursing of the patient. In the event of
a power failure, the nurse must know how to work the
machine manually.

A patient on a mechanical ventilator requires the
following observations:
1. *Chest movement.* If the chest wall is not rising in
   time with the respirator's action, the tubing should
   be checked to see that it has not become disconnected. If the patient breathes spontaneously out of
   phase with the ventilator, the nurse should notify

the doctor who may consider discontinuing the use of the ventilator or giving a muscle paralysing agent to allow the ventilator to fully control respiration.

2. *Colour.* If cyanosis occurs the doctor must be informed.

3. *Blood pressure, pulse and respiration rates* are noted.

4. *Volume of air* given at each inspiration is noted.

5. *The expired volume of air per minute* is noted, together with the positive and negative pressures of the machine.

   If there is a *rising positive pressure*, obstruction may be present or the patient may be attempting to breathe spontaneously. Tubing should be checked for kinking. Water which collects in the loops of the tubing should be emptied. Suction should be applied to the trachea. If no cause is found, the doctor must be notified.

   If there is a *falling positive pressure*, all tubing must be checked for air leaks, particularly at connections and at the cuff of the endotracheal or tracheostomy tube.

6. *Pupil reaction.* The nurse should remember that muscle paralysing agents such as tubocurarine do not affect pupil reaction.

7. The *temperature* within the humidifier and the *level of sterile distilled water* must be checked and maintained at normal.

8. The *observations related to the general nursing care* of the patient will of course be made, and particular attention should be given to the *pressure areas* and to the *mouth*.

Other respirators, originally known as 'iron lungs', work on the same principle as physiological respiration. They are also known as 'negative-positive pressure respirators'. A large pump rhythmically withdraws air from the cabinet in which the patient is enclosed and then allows it to return. In this way air is alternately drawn in to the patient's lungs and then expelled, as in normal respiration. Although these models have been much improved in recent years, it is thought that the negative pressure inside the cabinet tends to draw blood away from the heart. Nursing treatments are also difficult to carry out as the patient must be completely enclosed from the neck downwards inside the cabinet. If bulbar paralysis develops, the saliva which collects in the nasopharynx, due to an inability to swallow, can be sucked into the lungs as the pressure changes from negative to positive and could ultimately asphyxiate the patient.

Oxygen Tents

The tent method of administering oxygen is often used for children. There are several different types in use. Essentially the tent consists of a canopy of transparent plastic material mounted on a wheeled frame with metal stretchers to support the head of the canopy. There are openings in the canopy through which the nurse's arms can reach the patient to give any necessary attention. Cooling of the air inside the tent is achieved by passing the air through an ice box or through a refrigeration unit, and in some types of tent the carbon dioxide is removed by passing the air through soda-lime.

Before erection of the tent, a full cylinder of oxygen should be obtained, ready for use (see p. 34), and also, where necessary, a supply of ice. A wall thermometer will also be needed, to record the temperature inside the tent, which is usually maintained at 18–21°C.

If the tent has an ice cabinet, the ice is broken into

pieces about the size of a man's fist and the ice container filled to capacity. About 1 m of rubber tubing is then connected to the water outlet of the ice cabinet and a pail is placed under the rubber drainpipe. The ice cabinet is raised so that it will be clear of the ground when the canopy is fitted; the lid of the cabinet must be securely fastened otherwise there will be a leak of oxygen. A water seal is provided in the cabinet to prevent oxygen leaking through the drainpipe. The head of the canopy must be securely attached to the openings provided on the ice cabinet. This is done by means of rubber inserts or rubber corrugated tubing.

The back of the canopy has a nozzle marked 'oxygen inlet' to which the rubber tubing from the cylinder regulator is attached. This should be done, and the flow adjusted to 5 litres a minute, before the canopy is placed over the patient. The temperature control should be set to 'cold'. Two people are needed to fit the canopy over the patient's bed. The height of the tent and cabinet must be adjusted so that the head of the canopy will be about 15 cm above the patient's head. The skirt of the canopy is lifted and spread out so that it covers the bed and can be tucked in all round. In most tents the openings of the canopy have zip fasteners or are sealed by rolling them up and securing the flaps with bulldog clips.

As the tent is set up the oxygen flow should be turned on until the needle of the litre gauge registers 'flush'. This full flow is allowed to continue for about five minutes, then the flow is reduced to the dosage ordered, which may be from 4 to 8 litres per minute. All patients, and children in particular, should be provided with a hand bell. Many feel a sense of claustrophobia or isolation, so that, where possible, continuous or very frequent observation should be employed.

Some tents have an electric motor incorporated which circulates the oxygen, allows greater control of the temperature and improves the ventilation inside the tent.

When an oxygen tent is dismantled after use, the canopy should be mopped with a disinfectant solution and then washed with soap and water.

When high humidity conditions are required 'Humidair' type oxygen tents are very satisfactory.

Suction

Most wards are provided with wall-mounted suction machines. Small hand-operated bellows may be used in an emergency or whilst moving a patient but they are not as effective as a machine. The ideal position for the patient is with the head slightly extended; this prevents the catheter entering the oesophagus instead of the trachea when the swallowing reflex is still present. The patient's head is turned first to one side and then the other to introduce the catheter into each bronchus in turn; this avoids the natural tendency of the catheter to enter the right bronchus. The suction machine is turned on to the required pressure and the sterile catheter is connected to a Y connection on the tubing leading from the machine; the catheter should be handled with forceps or gloved hands. It is then introduced into the nasal passages and passed gently onwards until it reaches the excess secretions. At this point, the nurse covers the open end of the Y connection on the tubing and withdraws the catheter gently so that suction is only applied as the catheter is withdrawn. This prevents the mucosa adhering to the end. Failure to handle the catheter gently may result in bruising or even haemorrhage within the trachea. If the patient coughs during the procedure, the sputum expectorated must be aspirated. The nurse should observe and report on the nature of the sputum aspirated. Suction must not be prolonged because this causes discomfort to the patient. If suction by this method is not satisfactory, bronchoscopy may be required.

If the suction apparatus is incorporated into an intermittent positive pressure machine, the suction must be switched off immediately after use as it affects the running of the respirator. Disposable catheters are discarded after use.

Oxygen with Tracheostomy

When a patient has had a tracheostomy performed he obviously cannot benefit from oxygen given by a face mask or nasal tubes.

A perspex collar is available which fits round the patient's neck over the tracheostomy tube (Oxygenaire). An opening in the front of the collar with a 'pear-drop' cover allows suction to be carried out with the collar in position. Perforations at the side of the collar permit the escape of expired air and also allow the patient to continue to breathe should the oxygen supply accidentally fail.

If the oxygen collar is not available then oxygen must be given through tubing connected to the opening of the tracheostomy tube.

Under certain circumstances the nursing staff will be instructed to deflate the cuff on the tracheostomy tube at regular intervals. The procedure should be as follows:

1. The patient's mouth should be cleansed and the machine then disconnected.
2. The suction catheter is introduced into the trachea and the cuff is deflated immediately afterwards.

3. Any secretions that may have trickled past the cuff are aspirated.
4. The machine is re-connected.
5. The cuff is reinflated after five minutes with just enough air to prevent leakage around it; over-inflation can cause damage to the trachea.

The nurse may be asked to introduce a measured amount of a specified fluid down the tracheostomy tube at specified times. After introducing the fluid, the plug is replaced and the patient is allowed three breaths. By manipulating the Y tube of the catheter, suction is then applied during withdrawal. It should be possible to introduce the fluid and to suck out thoroughly in about thirty seconds. It is important that the patient should not be left off a ventilation machine for longer periods than this.

Hyperbaric Oxygen

Special chambers or tanks are needed for the administration of oxygen which is raised to 2 or 3 atmospheres pressure so that the blood may become supersaturated with a high tension of dissolved oxygen. This technique may be used in carbon monoxide poisoning, gas gangrene, or myocardial infarction.

7
Fluid and Electrolyte Balance

In health, the amount of fluid in the body, and its composition, remain remarkably constant in spite of variations in intake, but in almost every case of serious illness or extensive surgery the balance can be gravely disturbed and may need restoring urgently. For this reason one of the nurse's most valuable contributions to the treatment of the patient is the accurate recording of all fluid intake and output on the fluid balance chart, and noting the volume, route and type of fluid involved.

Body Water Content

The total quantity of water in the adult body amounts to approximately 70% of the body weight. Two-thirds of the water is inside the cells (intracellular) and one-third is outside the cells (extracellular). Most of the extracellular water is contained in the blood plasma and the interstitial fluid (lymph) which bathes tissue cells. So for an adult weighing 70 kg, approximately 50 kg would be water. 1 kg of body fluid has a volume of roughly 1 litre, so 34 litres of this body fluid would lie in the intracellular compartment while 16 litres would be extracellular (see Figure 6). Approximately 5% of the total body weight is accounted for by the water content (about 3.5 litres) of the blood.

Electrolytes

Many substances are contained in solution in the body fluids. Some of these, such as glucose, provide food for the cells; others, such as urea, are the waste

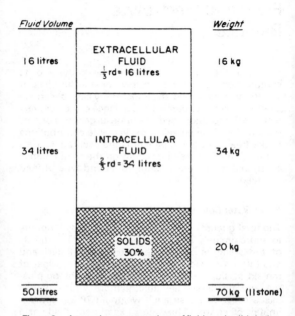

Figure 6. Approximate proportions of fluids and solids in the adult body

products of cell metabolism and must be removed. The interstitial fluid must be able to exchange with the blood plasma as well as with the intracellular fluid in order to transfer to the cell those substances that it needs and to clear waste substances from the cell into the blood.

Intracellular and extracellular fluids both contain salts in solution, the presence of which in the correct concentration is responsible for the interchange of material through the semi-permeable (differentially permeable) membrane which forms the cell boundary. These all-important salts form electrolytes, i.e. in solution they dissociate into electrically-charged particles, or ions. Some ions carry a positive charge and are known as cations, others are negatively charged and are called anions (see Figure 7).

The electrolytes in the extracellular fluid are mainly sodium and chloride, while the intracellular fluid contains mainly potassium and phosphate with a little chloride. The concentration of electrolytes is expressed in millimoles per litre, abbreviated to read mmol/litre (or mEq/litre, i.e. milli-equivalents per litre). ·

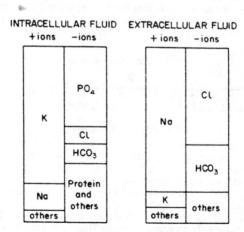

Figure 7. Comparison of electrolytes in the intracellular and extracellular fluids

The normal values of the common electrolytes found in the plasma are:

Bicarbonate (HCO_3)	21–32 mmol/litre
Chloride (Cl)	95–105 mmol/litre
Potassium (K)	3.8–5.0 mmol/litre
Sodium (Na)	136–148 mmol/litre
Phosphate (PO_4)	0.8–1.4 mmol/litre

Acid–Base Balance — the pH Scale

The pH formula gives the concentration of hydrogen ions in solution; acid solutions have a higher concentration of these ions than alkaline solutions. The pH scale runs from 0 to 14, with 7 representing neutrality (see Figure 8). The higher the hydrogen ion concentration the lower will be the reading, so if a solution gives a reading below 7 it is acid, if above 7 it is alkaline.

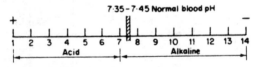

Figure 8. The pH scale

The maintenance of the normal pH of both the extracellular and intracellular fluids is another factor which governs the health of the cells. The extracellular fluid is normally slightly alkaline and has a pH value of 7.35–7.45. Intracellular fluid is slightly acid but its exact pH is not known.

The pH of both intracellular and extracellular fluids remains very constant in health. However, urine has a variable pH; although usually slightly acid, it can vary between 4.7 and 8. This is because one of the main functions of the kidneys is to maintain the normal pH value of the body fluids by excreting any excess of either acid or base (bicarbonate). The terms alkalosis and acidosis are used to indicate respectively that the blood contains an excess of base or acid.

Daily Requirements for Water and Electrolytes

An adult excretes about 1 litre of urine every 24 hours and also loses about 1 litre of water in the air expired from the lungs. Water is also lost through perspiration and in the water content of the faeces. An adult therefore needs to take in about 2 litres of fluid every 24 hours to replace this loss. No harm results from excessive intake of fluid in health as the kidneys are well able to dispose of unwanted fluid. If there is an increase in the loss of water, for example due to heavy perspiration, this will normally be made good immediately; the individual will feel thirsty and drink freely.

The minimum daily requirement of sodium is well exceeded by the average dietary intake of 5 g per day. Sodium deficit in health is unlikely since common table salt is often added either to our cooking or to our food. Potassium and other salts are also present in adequate amounts in the normal diet. In illness, however, both water and salt often need to be given intravenously. Accurate fluid balance recordings and frequent estimations of blood electrolyte levels are required if fluid and electrolyte replacement therapy is to succeed.

Fluid and Electrolyte Disturbances

In practice, disturbances in water content, electrolytes, and acid-base balance usually occur simultaneously.

For clarity of description, however, it is convenient to consider the most important factors and their appropriate treatment separately.

Water

Water depletion Excessive loss of water or diminished intake, or a combination of both, may lead to water depletion. Loss of fluid may not be obvious; in intestinal obstruction, for example, large quantities of fluid can collect in the distended intestine, in addition to that lost by vomiting. Depletion due to lowered intake is particularly liable to occur in comatose or semi-comatose patients.

Lack of water is characterised by thirst, dry mouth and tongue and decreased urinary output (oliguria). In severe cases, the patient has a pale, anxious face with sunken eyes, the extremities are cold and may be cyanosed, the skin loses its elasticity, and in infants the fontanelle is depressed. The pulse rate is usually rapid and the blood pressure low.

Water depletion can be corrected by giving the patient calculated amounts of oral or intragastric fluids, if the patient's condition permits. Alternatively the doctor may prescribe an intravenous infusion of 5% glucose solution in water. In those cases where electrolyte disturbance accompanies water depletion, electrolyte replacement therapy must be monitored by electrolyte estimations.

Water excess or 'intoxication' Water excess may be caused by the administration of large amounts of fluids to patients with poor urinary output. The effects of water intoxication are due to increased tension within the cells.

The clinical manifestations are mental confusion, convulsions, and coma. Muscle cramps may also occur. Chronic intoxication produces oedema of the lungs and the systemic circulation.

Such intoxication can be prevented by recording the volume of intake over a 24-hour period and relating the total figure to normal physiological needs. Those patients who are prone to oedema may be restricted to 1 litre of fluid plus the volume of the urinary output over the previous 24 hours. Severe oedema can be treated by severe water restriction or the use of diuretics.

Sodium

Sodium depletion (hyponatraemia) Sodium depletion may occur as a result of prolonged vomiting, gastric or intestinal aspiration, wound drainage or diarrhoea. The polyuria of diabetes causes a considerable depletion of sodium, and in Addison's disease and some cases of chronic nephritis sodium depletion may be a marked feature.

Sodium depletion is characterized by loss of skin elasticity and low intraocular pressure, and in cases of severe depletion by low blood pressure, circulatory failure, apathy, confusion and shock.

Sodium loss can be made good by the administration of salt either by mouth or, more commonly, by intravenous infusion of normal (isotonic) saline 0.9% solution.

Sodium excess (hypernatraemia) Sodium excess may be present in cases of cardiac failure and in the nephrotic syndrome, or it may be produced by large doses of cortisone or intravenous infusions of saline given rapidly or in excessive amounts.

The effect of sodium excess is to cause oedema, which is most dangerous when it affects the lungs.

Treatment is related to the cause.

Potassium

Potassium depletion (hypokalaemia)   Lack of potassium may be due to a low intake, persistent vomiting, gastric aspiration, Cushing's syndrome, diarrhoea, chronic renal disease, diabetic ketosis, excessive administration of cortisone or diuretics or occasionally to an adrenal tumour which is secreting aldosterone.

The chief manifestations of potassium lack are muscular weakness, intestinal paralysis, and myocardial failure.

The deficiency is made good by replacement therapy using oral preparations of potassium chloride or potassium citrate mixture. Potassium may be also given intravenously; the rate of administration should not exceed 20 mmol per hour so that the potassium plasma level remains within the normal range of 3.8–5.0 mmol per litre.

Potassium excess (hyperkalaemia)   Potassium excess occurs in cases of anuria (no urine output) from any cause and in Addison's disease of the adrenal cortex.

Its effect is to produce listlessness, mental confusion, and numbness and tingling of the extremities. As the plasma potassium level rises, there is grave danger of cardiac arrest.

In any of the above conditions it is necessary to avoid giving potassium in any form, e.g. in citrus fruit drinks. The treatment of hyperkalaemia may involve fasting the patient. An intravenous infusion of 10% glucose with 50 units of insulin is given to induce transfer of the potassium from the blood to the intracellular fluid. Ion exchange resins such as Resonium A may be given orally. If the patient is in renal failure, haemodialysis may be necessary.

Bicarbonate

Changes in the bicarbonate (HCO_3) content of the plasma reflect disturbances in the acid–base balance of the body.

Acidosis In acidosis the pH of the blood falls. This may be due to the formation of acids (as in diabetic ketosis when ketones are produced, or shock and tissue anoxia when lactic acid is produced), to the administration of acid-forming substances such as salicylates, or to decreased excretion of acid metabolites due to renal failure. Acidosis can also result from excessive loss of sodium bicarbonate as, for example, in cases of severe diarrhoea. When due to one of the above causes, the fall in pH is known as *metabolic acidosis*. In chronic respiratory disease, such as chronic bronchitis or emphysema, acidosis can occur from retention of carbon dioxide; this is known as *respiratory acidosis*.

Non-respiratory acidosis causes hyperventilation, with deep sighing respirations — the 'acidotic breathing' seen in diabetic coma and uraemia — and leads to mental confusion and coma.

Treatment is based upon the underlying cause, i.e. insulin for diabetic ketosis, peritoneal dialysis or haemodialysis for uraemia, and intermittent oxygen therapy for chronic bronchitis.

Alkalosis In alkalosis there is an increase in the pH of the blood. Alkalosis may be due to excessive and prolonged administration of alkalis or to loss of hydrochloric acid from persistent vomiting or gastric aspiration, causing the amount of bicarbonate in the blood plasma to increase.

The clinical signs are anorexia, mental confusion, slow shallow breathing and sometimes tetany; long-standing alkalosis may produce renal failure.

The treatment is based upon the precipitating cause. The condition may also be treated with intravenous infusion of normal saline; if renal function is normal the kidneys will retain the chloride and excrete the excess bicarbonate with the sodium. Potassium deficiency usually complicates alkalosis and this needs to be corrected simultaneously with sodium chloride treatment.

8
Intravenous Therapy, Blood Transfusion and Dialysis

Replacement of large amounts of fluid or blood lost from the body or the correction of serious electrolyte imbalance is most rapidly and accurately dealt with by the introduction of a suitable solution directly into the venous circulation. The composition of some of the proprietary intravenous solutions commonly used is given in Table III. The solutions are individually pre-scribed and the treatment monitored by frequent blood examinations. Nutrients may also be given intravenously. In all cases the rate of flow prescribed must be carefully maintained, and accurate records kept of the fluid given by this and any other route and of the patient's urinary output. Should the doctor prescribe say, 500 ml. of 0.9% normal (isotonic) saline 4-hourly, the nurse must be able to calculate the required rate of flow in order to control the amount of fluid passing through the drip chamber of the in-travenous set. The necessary formula is:

$$\frac{\text{prescribed volume (millilitres)}}{\text{prescribed time (hours)}} \times \frac{\text{drops per millilitre}}{60}$$

Since 1 ml of normal saline contains about 15 drops, for 500 ml 4-hourly the drip rate is:

$$\frac{500}{4} \times \frac{15}{60} = 31.25$$

which is approximately 30 drops/minute.

For normal saline and dextrose, 1 ml contains, on average, 15–17 drops. However, this may not be true for large molecular solutions such as Intralipid, blood, plasma and other protein fractions, so the outer wrapping should always be checked for the number of drops per millilitre recommended by the manu-facturers.

Table III.   Proprietary intravenous solutions

Solution	Electrolyte (mmol/litre)							Energy value* (kJ/litre)
	Na	K	Ca	Mg	Cl	HCO$_3$	pH	
Dextrose 5%	—	—	—	—	—	—	4	—
Dextrose 10%	—	—	—	—	—	—	4	1580
Sodium chloride 0.9%	150	—	—	—	150	—	5.5	—
Sodium chloride 0.9% with dextrose 5%	150	—	—	—	150	—	4	790
Darrow's solution†	121	35	—	—	103	—	6.5	—
Ringer's solution	147	4.5	2	—	156	—	5.5	—
Sodium lactate (6M)†	167	—	—	—	—	—	6.5	—
Hartmann's solution†	131	5	2	—	111	—	6.6	—
Laevulose 5%	—	—	—	—	—	—	4	790
Mannitol 10%	—	—	—	—	—	—	6	—
Sodium bicarbonate 4.2%	501	—	—	—	—	501	7.5	—
Sodium chloride 0.9% with potassium 0.15%	150	20	—	—	170	—	5.5	—

Sodium chloride 0.9% with potassium 0.2%	150	27	—	—	170	—	5·5	—
Sodium chloride 0.9% with potassium 0.3%	150	40	—	—	190	—	5·5	—
(Potassium is also available in proprietary dextrose solutions)								
Multiple electrolyte solution‡	140	5	—	1·5	98	—	5·5	80
Dextrans (plasma-expanders)								
6% Dextran 70 in 0.9% sodium chloride	150	—	—	—	150	—	5·5	—
10%Dextran 40 in 5% dextrose	—	—	—	—	—	—	5·5	790

* 4·2kJ = approx. 1 kilocalorie (Calorie)

† Lactate = 53 mmol/litre (Darrow's); 167 mmol/litre (sodium lactate); 29 mmol/litre (Hartmann's).

‡ Also contains 27 mmol/litre acetate and 23 mmol/litre gluconate.

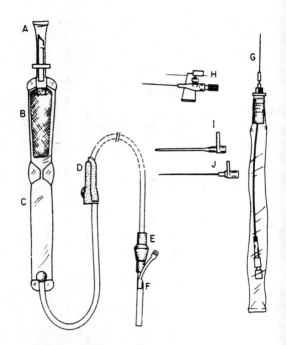

Figure 9. Disposable giving set (without air inlet)
A   Sealed needle for insertion into Viaflex bag.
B   Filter chamber.
C   Drip chamber — must never be allowed to become empty.
D   Control clamp — used to control the rate of flow.
E   Rubber seal for injecting additional drugs.
F   Connection to intravenous needle/catheter.
G-J   Examples of intravenous needles/catheters (H: Viggo; I and J: Branulas).

The Giving Set

A giving set is shown in Figure 9. Air is expelled from the tubing by running the infusion fluid through it before the set is connected to the patient. The apparatus for intravenous infusion and transfusion supplied by commercial firms is always disposable. It should never be used if the seal is broken. The outer wrapping should be checked for an expiry date.

Parenteral Feeding

The composition and calorific content of some proprietary solutions commonly used in parenteral (intravenous) feeding are given in Table IV. Since parenteral feeding carries some risks, the patient should be weighed daily if possible, and fluid balance charts should be completed with particular care. Because some of these infusions have a high sugar content, urine analysis for glucose may have to be done 4-hourly. A 24-hour urine specimen may have to be collected for urea and electrolytes, and daily assessment of blood glucose levels will be required to determine the nutritional regimen on a daily basis. Since the administration of parenteral feeding solutions is highly irritant to the walls of the superficial veins, a central venous catheter is commonly used for this type of therapy.

Central Venous Pressure

The physiological changes in patients with sudden severe shock and a decreased venous return to the heart can be monitored by taking measurements of the central venous pressure. A long catheter is passed, preferably into the right antecubital vein, and threaded

Table IV. Solutions commonly used in parenteral (intravenous) feeding

Preparation	Contents	Energy Content (kJ/litre)	K	Na	Ca	Cl	Glucose	Fat	Glycerol	Sorbitol
					mmol/litre				g/litre	
Glucose 10%	Dextrose 10%	1700	—	—	—	—	100	—	—	—
Glucose 50%	Dextrose 50%	8610	—	—	—	—	500	—	—	—
Vamin glucose	Synthetic amino acids	1050	20	50	—	55	—	—	—	—
Vamin N	Synthetic amino acids	1050	20	50	2·5	55	—	—	—	—
Aminosol	Caesin hydrolysate	1390	0·6	160	—	130	—	—	—	—
Aminoplex	Synthetic amino acids + sorbitol 10% + ethanol 5%	4200	15	35	—	62	—	—	—	125
Aminoplex 14	Synthetic amino acids	1430	30	35	—	81	—	—	—	—
Intralipid 10%	Soya bean oil + fractionated egg + lecithin 12g	4200	—	—	—	—	—	100	12	—
Intralipid 20%	Soya bean oil + fractionated egg + lecithin 12g	8400	—	—	—	—	—	200	25	—

into the major veins of the upper arm towards the superior vena cava and right atrium. The normal venous pressure in the right atrium varies between 4 and 14 mmH$_2$O. If the pressure recorded on the attached manometer is below 4 mmH$_2$O then the patient is hypovolaemic. If the pressure is above 14 mmH$_2$O then it is possible that the patient is being over-transfused. Such measurements are repeated frequently in right-sided heart failure, to monitor the results of intensive infusion therapy, or in patients requiring intensive parenteral feeding.

Intravenous Drugs

Qualified nurses specially trained in the technique of giving intravenous injections may inject drugs directly into a vein; otherwise only a doctor may perform this duty. Drugs given intravenously are rapidly absorbed. As an alternative to injection directly into a vein, they may be given intermittently by being added to an infusion bag or bottle, or continuously by motorised infusion pump.

The following are examples of drugs commonly given intravenously:

Potassium chloride—using manufactured solutions containing potassium (see page 56).

Heparin—either intermittently or continuously using the motorized infusion pump.

Lignocaine—preferably administered using manufactured infusion solutions.

Antibiotics—benzylpenicillin, ampicillin, cloxacillin, flucloxacillin, carbenicillin, cephaloridine and cephalothin, gentamicin, tetracyclines, fusidic acid and lincomycin. Certain combinations of antibiotics and infusion fluids may be contra-indicated; the advice of the hospital pharmacy should always be sought if the drug instructions are not clear.

Corticosteroids—either intermittently or continuously. The drugs which are specifically for intravenous use are clearly labelled by the manufacturer.

Cytotoxic drugs—invariably prescribed for continuous infusion by motorized infusion pump.

Transfusion Fluids

The usual indications for transfusion of blood, plasma or plasma substitutes are haemorrhage, burns, major surgery and severe anaemia. The standard transfusion fluids provided by the Blood Transfusion Services of the United Kingdom are:

1. Whole blood.
2. Concentrated suspension of red blood cells.
3. Dried plasma (reconstituted with sterile distilled water).
4. Packed cells.
5. Fractionated cellular components.

There are also a number of plasma substitutes available from commercial sources, e.g. dextran 10%, which are also referred to as 'plasma volume expanders'.

Blood Groups

Transfusion of blood from one person to another carries great risks unless it can be proved that the blood of the donor is compatible with the blood of the recipient. Every individual has antibodies in his blood which react against 'foreign' proteins including, in some cases, the proteins in the blood cells of another human being. The effect of these antibodies is to cause agglutination, or clumping, of the red blood cells. Sometimes, however, the individual will not produce antibodies in response to foreign red cells entering his blood stream and in this case the blood of the donor is said to be compatible with that of the recipient; both these individuals belong to the same blood group. Human blood is, therefore, classified according to the type of red cell present. The most important classifications are known as the ABO and the Rhesus (Rh) systems. The ABO and Rh groups of the donor and recipient must be compatible. As a further check, since sub-groups may also be present, and because people acquire agglutinating antibodies in addition to the 'natural' antibodies, it is necessary to carry out direct tests matching the recipient's blood against the blood to be donated.

ABO system (Figure 10)   Human blood falls into one of four ABO categories, A, B, AB or O. Groups AB and B are comparatively rare in European populations, most of whose members belong to either the A or the O group.

Group A.   This group has A antigens in the red cells and anti-B antibodies in the plasma.

Group B.   This group has B antigens in the red cells and anti-A antibodies in the plasma.

Group AB.   This group has both A and B antigens in the red cells but the plasma contains neither anti-A nor anti-B antibodies.

Group O.   This group has no A or B antigens in the red cells but has both anti-A and anti-B antibodies in the plasma.

Group A, therefore, cannot receive blood from Group B as the A group contains anti-B antibodies. Group B similarly cannot receive blood from Group A.

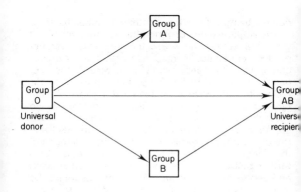

Figure 10. Blood group compatibility – the ABO system

Group AB has neither anti-A nor anti-B antibodies and therefore, theoretically, can receive blood from all other groups ('universal recipient').

Group O has both anti-A and anti-B antibodies and can therefore receive only Group O blood. As Group O red cells carry neither A nor B antigens, this group can give to all other ABO groups as the red cells of O group will not be agglutinated by the recipient's plasma. Group O is sometimes referred to as the 'universal donor group' and may in cases of extreme emergency be given to a patient without awaiting the results of full cross-matching tests. In practice this is rarely done.

Rhesus group system   The Rhesus, or Rh group, was given this name as it was found that the same system of antibodies was present in the blood of the rhesus monkey. In this system the most important factor is labelled 'D'; the majority of Europeans have this D substance in their blood and are therefore described as Rh positive. About 15% of the population, however, do not have the Rh factor D and are said to be Rh negative. Transfusion of Rh positive blood to a Rh negative individual can be dangerous, since the Rh negative blood will produce antibodies to destroy the transfused cells. The effect of a first transfusion may be slight, but the individual becomes sensitive to the D factor and further transfusions with Rh positive blood may produce a serious reaction. A similar reaction can take place in the fetus when the mother's blood is Rh negative but that of the fetus is Rh positive. The maternal blood then produces antibodies which enter the fetal circulation via the placenta and destroy the fetal red blood cells. The fetus may die or, if surviving to term, may be born with a severe type of haemolytic jaundice. Since sensitivity to the D factor takes some time to develop, it is unusual for this reaction to occur in a first pregnancy unless the Rh negative woman has been transfused with Rh positive blood.

The units of whole blood supplied by the Blood Transfusion Services are labelled to show the ABO and Rh groups, the date of collection of the blood from the donor and the date after which the blood is unfit for transfusion. Each unit of stored whole blood contains 120 ml of an anticoagulant solution. Stocks for hospital blood banks and sterilized disposable giving sets are supplied by regional centres of the Blood Transfusion Services. Mobile units from these centres also arrange donor sessions at hospitals and other convenient places, where blood is collected to maintain the stocks held at the regional centre.

Management of Transfusion

In all cases where blood transfusion is needed, 5 ml of the patient's blood is sent to a laboratory for grouping and direct cross-matching tests with a sample of the blood to be transfused. Any error in the labelling of this specimen or the accompanying laboratory form could lead to incompatible blood being given.

The correct blood for the individual patient is then labelled with his full name, ward name, and case note number, and a statement that the blood is compatible is signed. The particulars on the bottle or Viaflex unit of blood should be checked when the blood is removed from the blood bank in order to ensure that the right blood is given to the right patient. Almost every case of incompatible blood transfusion is due to an administrative error, such as incorrect labelling or failure to check the label carefully. The nurse should be particularly careful when there are two patients in the same ward with the same name.

Stored blood must be kept at a temperature between 4 and 6°C in a thermostatically controlled refrigerator. It should never be cooled below 4°C or heated in any way. Bottles or plastic units of blood are always carefully handled to avoid shaking the contents, but it is permissible to mix the blood gently if the cells have settled to the bottom.

Whole blood may be used up to 21 days after withdrawal from the donor, provided that it is properly stored. Red cell suspensions must be used within 24 hours of preparation.

Requirements for Transfusion

The following equipment is required:
1. Disposable giving set.

2. Sterile pack containing swabs, paper towels and disposable gallipots.
3. Skin cleansing lotion.
4. Sphygmomanometer cuff or tourniquet to distend superficial veins.
5. Adhesive strapping and scissors.
6. Protective polythene sheeting for the bedclothes.

The same equipment is used for both transfusion and infusion. The introduction of a needle or catheter into a vein is an aseptic technique. Where intravenous therapy is to be continued for several days, a length of fine polythene tubing (Intracath) may be introduced into the superficial vein and threaded into the deeper veins; this technique reduces the risk of superficial venous irritation or thrombophlebitis.

Occasionally the doctor may have to cut down into a vein in a patient with severe circulatory collapse. The instruments for this procedure are supplied by either the Central Sterile Supply Department (CSSD) or Theatre Sterile Unit (TSU), and may be stored on the resuscitation trolley. The *cut down set* contains:

1. Scapel or knife handle and blade.
2. One pair of toothed fine dissecting forceps.
3. One pair of non-toothed fine dissecting forceps.
4. One pair of fine pointed scissors.
5. Two fine artery forceps.
6. Aneurysm needle.
7. Catgut or nylon size 0/0.
8. Two curved skin needles and sutures.
9. Intravenous cannula or fine polythene tubing with adaptor.
10. Hypodermic syringe, needles and local anaesthetic.

Clear instructions on the setting up of apparatus are issued on the back of each container and these must be followed carefully. The nurse is responsible for assisting the doctor in this aseptic technique and adjusting the clamp to control the required rate of flow.

The intravenous needle or catheter should be kept in position with adhesive strapping, with the arm or lower limb resting comfortably on a protected pillow. In the case of infants, young children or very restless patients it may be necessary to splint the limb. The bandage used to fix the splint must be taken over bony prominences in order to avoid the risk of obstructing the venous circulation. The veins of the scalp may be used in infants instead of the veins in the arms or legs.

Rate of Flow of Blood

For slow transfusions the recommended rate of flow is 40 drops per minute. Rapid transfusions may be needed to replace a severe and sudden loss of blood; in such cases one or more units of blood may be given as rapidly as the blood will flow into the vein. In extreme urgency intra-arterial transfusions have been given but this technique is now rarely used. For the rate of flow of infusions see p. 55.

Changing Bottles

Blood is usually collected from the hospital blood bank unit by unit as it is required. After careful checking of the labels and the patient's identity wrist band, the unit of blood is placed by the bedside. When the level of the transfusing blood is just above the neck of the bottle, the clamp is turned to seal off the tubing of the giving set. The plastic seal of the new unit of blood, which will be pierced by the needle, is swabbed with an antiseptic solution. The new unit of blood is then hung alongside the transfused unit and the piercing needle transferred from the old to the new unit of blood as cleanly as possible. The needle must not be allowed to touch the outside or the edge of either blood container during this procedure. The tubing clamp is then released and the transfusion continued at the prescribed rate. The empty bottle or plastic blood container should be kept for 24 hours before disposal.

The disposable blood pack unit has the advantage over the glass bottle that plasma, platelets, anti-D factor and antihaemophilic globulin can all be safely transfused using the disposable pack.

Risks Associated with Blood Transfusions and Infusions

The introduction of large volumes of blood or fluid into the blood stream can give rise to *cardiac and respiratory distress* as a result of overloading the circulatory system. The danger is greatest when large quantities of fluid are rapidly introduced, but problems can arise even with a slow transfusion, particularly in the elderly with weakened heart muscle or chronic anaemia. Signs which should be watched for and reported to the doctor immediately are:

1. Rising pulse rate.
2. Laboured breathing.
3. Cough.
4. Distended neck veins.
5. Oedema.

A fluid intake/output chart should always be kept for patients receiving parenteral fluids.

Reaction to the transfusion may occur soon after the transfusion has commenced. A severe reaction may be due to incompatibility of the blood causing haemolysis in the recipient's blood stream. The symptoms are shivering and rise of pulse and temperature; the patient may complain of severe pain in the lumbar region. *The transfusion must be stopped at once.* There is great danger of kidney damage with subsequent suppression of urine formation and renal failure.

A *pyrexial reaction* due to the introduction of foreign protein into the recipient's blood stream can give rise to rigors, fever, and an increased pulse rate. In this case the rate of the transfusion should be slowed down, chlorpheniramine 4 mg orally is occasionally prescribed to overcome this pyrexial reaction; if this is unsuccessful the transfusion must be stopped.

Thrombosis of the vein is not uncommon. It may be limited in extent and cause little trouble, but if it is extensive there is considerable pain in the limb and there may be a rise in the patient's temperature. The transfusion may have to be stopped and a hot application or an evaporating lotion may be ordered for the relief of pain.

A *haematoma* may form at the site of the transfusion as a result of the needle becoming dislodged from the vein and the blood being extravasated into the surrounding tissues. The transfusion must be stopped and the limb elevated. An injection of hyaluronidase may be given into the swollen area. If the haematoma occurs on the outer aspect of the arm or elbow the arteries supplying the forearm may be compressed; a regular careful count should be taken of the radial pulse, and the colour, feeling and peripheral temperature of the fingers and hand should be noted.

Sepsis may occur at the site of the infusion. This is more likely to occur when a cannula is tied into a vein than with the use of an intravenous needle or polythene tubing.

Air embolism is a rare occurrence but one which must be borne in mind. It is prevented by ensuring that air is expelled from the tubing before the transfusion is started and that the bottle or Viaflex unit is not allowed to become empty. The limb into which the transfusion is running should *never* be raised above the level of the patient's heart; if the bottle should run out, air will be sucked in. Pressure should not be used to push blood in at a faster rate but if necessary the level of the bottle can be raised. The patient with an embolism may complain of a variety of sensory disturbances, such as tingling in the fingers, and may collapse. The immediate treatment is to lower the patient's head and inform the doctor.

Difficulty in maintaining the flow of blood may be due to one of several causes:

1. Spasm of the vein. This may be overcome by gently warming the limb or stroking along the vein above the site of the injection.
2. Kinking or compression of the tubing. This possibility is easily checked up on by examining the tubing.
3. The needle may become dislodged. An attempt may be made to alter the position of the needle by gently lifting the mount to depress the point. This may be successful, but if the needle has punctured the wall of the vein, the transfusion will have to be stopped and, if necessary, started again using a different vein.
4. An airlock may block the flow of blood from the bag or bottle. This should not occur if due care is taken to expel all air from the delivery tubing before connecting it to the needle or cannula. If, however, an airlock should be present the apparatus must be disconnected from the needle and the blood

allowed to run freely through the tubing before it is again connected to the intravenous needle.

Prolonged intravenous infusion, particularly in the elderly, may lead to a *confused state* due to a shortage of vitamin B. If this is the case, Parentrovite can be administered via the infusion.

Intravenous Therapy in Babies and Children

The kidneys of babies and children are not as physiologically effective as those of adults and they are susceptible to acid-base upsets. For this reason intravenous fluids are given with caution and accurate observations are extremely important throughout the infusion. The electrolyte solutions given vary according to the degree of dehydration and the baby's condition.

Subcutaneous Infusion

In cases of dehydration, particularly in babies, it is possible to give fluid, usually saline or 5% dextrose, via the subcutaneous route, either intermittently or continuously, using hyaluronidase (Hyalase) to aid rapid absorption. The main value of this route is that a doctor is not required to administer the fluid. However, absorption is not so effective.

Dialysis

The need for dialysis arises in certain cases of acute disturbance of the electrolyte and fluid balance of the body following loss of kidney function, and when other measures have been ineffectual.

Dialysis works on the principle that if two solutions of different composition are separated by a membrane which is permeable to the small molecules in the solutions, these will cross the membrane until their concentration is equal on the two sides. Applied clinically, this means that dialysis can occur between the patient's blood and interstitial fluid (containing an excessive amount of waste products) and a specially prepared electrolyte solution (the dialysis fluid), using the peritoneum as the permeable membrane. Waste products pass into the dialysing fluid, which is then removed and replaced by a fresh supply.

In haemodialysis, blood is drawn out of the body and dialysed in a special machine (the artificial kidney) before being returned.

Where there is a rapid rise in blood urea and potassium, haemodialysis is more effective than peritoneal dialysis, mainly because the procedure takes less time. This method, however, requires the constant attention of experienced medical, nursing and technical staff as well as expensive and more bulky equipment.

Peritoneal Dialysis

Peritoneal dialysis can be undertaken in a ward, although a side ward is preferable. The equipment consists of a sterile disposable peritoneal catheter with a metal stylet for introduction and a giving set combined with a sterile plastic bag (or bottle) for collection of returning fluid. The dialysing fluid is contained in sterile plastic bags or in bottles. Proprietary equipment supplied by manufacturers give instructions and diagrams for aid in assembly.

The patient's bladder is emptied and the anterior abdominal wall prepared as for surgery. The semi-recumbent position is usually adopted. Under a local anaesthetic the catheter is introduced into the peritoneum slightly below the umbilicus in the midline. If an incision has been made, a skin suture may be required. The appropriate clips are adjusted. The warmed dialysing fluid is then run in to the peritoneal space as fast as it will go, taking about 10 minutes. Most patients will tolerate the introduction of two litres. The fluid remains in the peritoneal sac for roughly 20 to 30 minutes. The clips are then organized to allow it to run out into the collecting bag. Some doctors advise a firm abdominal binder to facilitate drainage. The drainage period should be limited to a maximum of 40 minutes and during the early stages it is usual for the volume of fluid run out to be less than that run in. With later exchanges a negative fluid balance is achieved. Failure to drain off sufficient fluid may lead to systemic overloading and/or pulmonary oedema. Blood pressure and fluid balance recordings must therefore be kept throughout. Defects in drainage can arise from catheter blockage due to deposition of fibrin. This may be controlled by adding 500 units of heparin per litre of dialysing fluid, hourly if necessary.

Microscopy and culture of the fluid may be ordered and some doctors prefer the addition of an antibiotic as a safeguard against infection. The protein content of the fluid must also be checked. Plasma may be ordered if the blood pressure falls.

Physiotherapy plays an important part in the prevention of pulmonary complications. Good nursing care, support and observation, together with aseptic technique throughout, add to the safety and effectiveness of this treatment.

Patients can be taught to control their own dialysis programme and maintain their independence if they are mentally and physically capable of doing so. This is known as Continuous Ambulatory Peritoneal Dialysis (CAPD). The patient is taught how to handle a permanent peritoneal catheter and its connections in a sterile manner. The patient is responsible for infusing the dialysis fluid into the peritoneal cavity in a given time, allowing time for exchange of molecules to occur, and then draining off the fluid. Prior to disconnecting the disposable tubing they may infuse a litre of dialysis fluid into the peritoneal cavity, which is retained for several hours until the next exchange is due. CAPD may be used by the patient while in hospital or if suitable conditions with supportive services are available, at home, until a donor kidney becomes available.

9
Administration of Controlled and Scheduled Drugs

Acts of Parliament control the supply and administration of many drugs. Most hospitals have supplemented the statutory requirements by additional rules. All drugs have an official name and it is recommended that this is used, but many are marketed by several different firms, each giving the drug its own proprietary name; to overcome this problem both the official and the proprietary name should be printed on the label of the drug container by the pharmacist. The Acts of particular concern to nurses are:

Misuse of Drugs Act (1971)
Poisons List and Rules Schedules I and IV (1972)
Therapeutic Substances Act (1956)

Misuse of Drugs Act (1971)

This Act is concerned with drugs which may give rise to addiction or dependence. They are commonly known as 'controlled drugs' and include, for example, opium and its derivatives such as papaveretum (Omnopon), morphine, diamorphine (heroin), pethidine and methadone.

The labels of containers for controlled drugs are marked CDA. In hospital controlled drugs must be kept in a locked cupboard used solely for this purpose. The key must be kept on the person of whoever is in charge of the ward or department. The drugs are ordered in a special printed book with carbon copies, and a receipt must be signed when they are delivered to the ward. The original requisition is kept in the pharmacy for two years. The custody of the drugs is the responsibility of the sister/charge nurse or her/his deputy, but the drug cupboards and records may be inspected at any time by the hospital pharmacist or a senior member of the nursing staff.

In most hospitals the regulations for administration of controlled drugs follow a meticulous routine whether the Kardex or a similar system operates, or the prescription is written on the patient's drug chart or in his notes. Two nurses (one of whom is registered or a senior enrolled nurse) check the prescription for:

1. The patient's full name.
2. The date.
3. The drug.
4. The dose.
5. The route.
6. The time of administration.
7. The doctor's signature.

After the required amount of drug has been removed from the cupboard the ampoules or tablets remaining are checked and recorded. Once the drug has been drawn into the syringe the details are checked once more with the prescription. The patient's identity and the administration of the drug are checked by both nurses at the patient's bedside and both sign the controlled drugs record book immediately afterwards. The drug chart and Kardex may also be signed and the time of administration recorded. No cancellation, obliteration or alteration to the records is permitted; corrections are made by marginal notation and are signed and witnessed.

Poisons List and Rules Schedules I and IV (1972)

This legislation is concerned with a large range of potentially dangerous or toxic drugs which are divided into 17 categories known as schedules. Each schedule is subject to special regulations, most of which involve the pharmacist. The nurse is chiefly concerned with Schedules I and IV.

The container of the scheduled drug must be labelled with a distinguishing mark or other indication which shows that it must be stored in a locked cupboard, reserved solely for poisons and other dangerous substances. The general practice in hospitals is for the controlled drugs cupboard to be contained within the poisons cupboard, each having its own key. Many of the cupboards are lit from within and a red light indicates that the door is open. If a ward drug trolley is used, it must be lockable and be securely parked when not in use, either in a lockable cupboard or fastened to the wall or floor.

Examples of Schedule 1 drugs: atropine, hyoscine, digoxin, cyclophosphamide, and barbiturate compounds. These are ordered in a separate book from the CDA drugs and are signed for on receipt.

Examples of Schedule IV drugs: diazepam, ephedrine, ergotamine, and chloral hydrate. These drugs are potentially harmful and most hospitals adopt a scheme of checking administration and recording of stock balance.

Therapeutic Substances Act (1956)

This Act is concerned with substances subject to the same restrictions as poisons. Examples are antibiotics, insulin, corticosteroids, vaccines, antitoxins and anticoagulants. Some of these drugs need to be stored in a locked refrigerator. The same pattern of checking and recording may apply as for scheduled drugs. Poisons which are for external use must be contained in a ribbed or fluted bottle which is distinguishable by touch and should be stored in a cupboard reserved solely for poisons and other dangerous substances. For safety, poisons for internal and external use are stored separately. Particular care should be taken with cupboards in sluice or pathology areas containing urinary reagents; these should be kept locked when not in use.

10
The Classification of Drugs

Anabolic agents   Tissue-building male sex hormones (androgens), prescribed to increase weight in patients suffering from wasting diseases or osteoporosis. Examples: methandienone (Dianabol), norethandrolone (Nilevar), nandrolone (Deca-Durabolin). See p. 106.

Anaesthetics   Drugs which produce insensibility to pain, either by general, regional, or local administration. Their general action causes a controllable but reversible loss of consciousness; the local action paralyses the nerve supply in the area of application. Examples of general anaesthetics are nitrous oxide and halothane (Fluothane) given by inhalation, and thiopentone sodium given by intravenous injection. Examples of topical local anaesthesia are lignocaine and cinchocaine (Nuperacine).

Analeptics   Drugs which stimulate both the respiratory and the central nervous system. They are usually prescribed in the event of respiratory failure due to overdose of hynoptic drugs when a respirator is not available. Examples: bemegride, pentetrazol (Leptazol) doxapram (Dopram), aminophylline, nikethamide.

Analgesics   Drugs which relieve pain. Examples: acetylsalicylic acid (aspirin), pethidine, morphine.

Antacids   Drugs which neutralize the acidity of the gastric juices. Examples: magnesium trisilicate, magnesium carbonate.

Anthelmintics   Drugs used to destroy or expel intestinal parasites. Examples: piperazine for roundworm and threadworm, bephenium (Alcopar) for hookworm.

Antibiotics Chemical substances, either synthetic or produced from living organisms, which inhibit the growth of or destroy organisms. Examples: penicillin, streptomycin.

Anticholinesterases Drugs which inhibit the enzyme cholinesterase which breaks down acetylcholine. These drugs allow acetylcholine to accumulate at the nerve endings and restore normal muscle tone. They are used mainly by anaesthetists to reverse the action of drugs used during surgery to produce muscle relaxation such as tubocurarine (Tubarine) and gallamine. They may also be used in the treatment of myasthenia gravis and glaucoma, and in cases of poisoning from certain agricultural insecticides. Examples: edrophonium (Tensilon), physostigmine (eserine), dyflos.

Anticoagulants Drugs which prevent blood from clotting in the blood vessels. Examples: heparin, phenindione (Dindevan), warfarin (Marevan), nicoumalone (Sinthrome).

Anticonvulsants Drugs which prevent and suppress abnormal brain rhythms which could induce convulsions. Examples: phenytoin (Epanutin), troxidone (Tridione) and phenobarbitone.

Antidepressants Drugs which relieve depression in the depressive illnesses. Examples: imipramine (Tofranil), amitriptyline (Tryptizol). (See also Monoamine oxidase inhibitors.)

Antihistamines   Drugs which neutralize the effects of histamines. Used for the treatment of angioneurotic oedema, urticaria and hay fever, and to prevent vomiting following anaesthesia or in travel sickness. Examples: mepyramine maleate (Anthisan), promethazine hydrochloride (Phenergan), promethazine theoclate (Avomine).

Antipyretics   Drugs which reduce the body temperature in a fever. Examples: acetylsalicylic acid (aspirin), quinine.

Antiseptics   Chemical substances which inhibit growth and reproduction of living micro-organisms. These drugs are also known as bacteriostatics. See p. 116.

Antispasmodics   Drugs relieving spasmodic contraction of involuntary muscles. Examples: atropine, glyceryl trinitrate, propantheline (Pro-Banthine).

Antithyroid drugs   Drugs which interfere with the production or manufacture of thyroxine by the thyroid gland. Examples: carbimazole (Neo-Mercazole), propylthiouracil. See p. 104.

Antitoxins   Chemical substances which neutralize bacterial toxins. See Sera, Toxoids.

Antiviral agents   Drugs used in the treatment of viral infections such as herpes simplex and herpes zoster. Example: idoxuridine (Herpid).

Aperients   Drugs which stimulate intestinal activity. Examples: senna, magnesium sulphate, bisacodyl (Dulcolax).

Bronchial dilators Drugs which cause relaxation of bronchial smooth muscle, thereby increasing vital capacity. They are given in the form of aerosol sprays for inhalation, sublingually, by injection or by mouth. Examples: isoprenaline, aminophylline, ephedrine, salbutamol (Ventolin) which is commonly used in asthma.

Carminatives Drugs which expel gas and relieve distension in the gastro-intestinal tract. Examples: magnesium carbonate mixture, oil of peppermint.

Contraceptives The contraceptive pill, commonly known as 'The Pill', is used in the prevention of pregnancy by inhibiting ovulation. It contains either oestrogen or progesterone in single or combined doses. Examples: Anovlar, Binovum, Conova, Ovulen, Norgestron. See p. 111.

Cytotoxic agents Drugs which act as a poison to certain living cells. Used in the treatment of malignant disease to destroy neoplastic cells. Examples: chlorambucil, methotrexate, vincristine, busulphan, cyclophosphamide, vinblastine.

Disinfectants Chemical substances which when used at a prescribed strength for a specific period of time will kill specified micro-organisms. Examples: chlorhexidine (Hibitane), gluteraldehyde solution. See p. 116.

Diuretics Drugs which increase the output of urine. Examples: hydrochlorothiazide, bendrofluazide, frusemide (Lasix), ethacrynic acid (Edecrin).

Emetics Drugs used to induce therapeutic emesis.

Examples: ipecacuanha syrup, apomorphine hydrochloride.

Expectorants Drugs increasing expectoration from the bronchial tree. Examples: potassium iodide, ammonium carbonate, ipecacuanha, bromhexine (Bisolvon).

Fertility drugs Drugs which increase the output of pituitary gonadotrophins which stimulate the maturation and endocrine activity of the ovarian follicle and the subsequent development of the corpus luteum. Example: Clomiphene (Clomid).

Hypnotics Drugs which induce sleep. Examples: amylobarbitone (Sodium Amytal), butobarbitone (Soneryl), nitrazepam (Mogadon).

Hypotensives Drugs which lower the blood pressure. Examples: propranolol (Inderal), methyldopa (Aldomet), guanethidine (Ismelin).

Monoamine oxidase inhibitors Drugs which act by causing amines normally present in the central nervous system to accumulate rather than be destroyed by enzymes, thus preventing certain depressive illnesses. Examples: phenalzine (Nardil), isocarboxazid (Marplan). MAO inhibitors have many other biochemical actions when taken in conjunction with other drugs, alcohol, or certain foods, such as strong cheese. Advice must be sought in relation to the patient's diet and the use of other drugs when MAO drugs are being administered.

Mucolytics Drugs which reduce the viscosity of bronchial secretions so easing expectoration. Examples: bromhexine (Bisolvon), acetylcysteine (Airbron), methylcysteine (Visclair), carbocisteine (Mucodyne).

Muscle relaxants   Drugs used, usually in combination with anaesthetics, to produce complete muscle relaxation which is independent of the depth of anaesthesia. Example: suxamethonium (Scoline).

Mydriatics   Drugs which dilate the pupil of the eye. Examples: atropine, homatropine.

Miotics   Drugs which contract the pupil of the eye, e.g. physostigmine, pilocarpine.

Narcotics   Drugs which depress the central nervous system, e.g. hypnotics and sedatives.

Prostaglandins   Prostaglandins are fatty acids with hormone-like actions which occur naturally in the body. They are also manufactured synthetically. Their principal known effect is on smooth muscle within the body, e.g. that of the respiratory, uterine and vascular systems. Prostaglandins are prescribed mainly to induce abortion or labour. Aspirin taken as medication is known to interfere with the natural synthesis of prostaglandins, which suggests that prostaglandins may be responsible for some of the inflammatory disorders that aspirin relieves.

Purgatives   Drugs which stimulate bowel action; the term is usually applied to those which have a drastic action. See Aperients (p. 82).

Sera   Serum is prepared from the blood of human beings who have suffered from a particular disease, or from animals, usually horses, who are given a vaccine or toxoid to stimulate the production of the appropriate antibodies or antitoxins. It is used to give protection from specific diseases when the need is urgent. This form of passive immunity can be provided in a matter of minutes but lasts only for a period of weeks since the serum contains proteins foreign to the human body. These can cause severe reactions in susceptible people. Sera may be used to give protection in the following diseases: anthrax, botulinus, gas gangrene, rabies and rubella (German measles). In persons susceptible to anti-tetanus serum an ovine serum (obtained from sheep) is available. See p. 95.

Toxoids   Liquids containing treated toxins which, when introduced into the body, stimulate active immunity against certain specific infections caused by bacterial toxins, e.g. diphtheria and tetanus. For persons susceptible to antitetanus toxoid, a human anti-immunoglobulin is available. See p. 95.

Tranquillizers   Drugs which reduce nervous tension without causing sleep. Examples: diazepam (Valium), chlordiazepoxide (Librium).

Vaccines   Suspensions of dead, living or attentuated micro-organisms or their toxins which, when introduced into the human body, stimulate active immunity against a specific infection. Diseases against which vaccination gives protection include typhoid fever (TAB), tuberculosis (BCG), poliomyelitis, tetanus, cholera, whooping cough and measles. See immunization table (p. 95).

11
Pharmaceutical Preparations

Capsules Drugs, usually either oily or nauseous preparations, enclosed in gelatine envelopes. Examples: chlordiazepoxide (Librium), halibut-liver oil.

Collodions Solutions of cellulose in alcohol and ether used to give a protective coating on the skin and over small dressings. Examples: flexible collodion, salicylic acid collodion.

Creams Semi-solid emulsions, usually made up with distilled water or liquid paraffin, for external application. Examples: zinc oxide, hydrocortisone.

Ear-drops Liquid for application to the external auditory meatus. Examples: sodium bicarbonate solution, Cerumol.

Elixirs Strong extracts of drugs usually made up with syrup and flavouring agents. Example: Brompton Cocktail. This is an oral mixture of chloroform, morphine, cocaine, gin, and honey, based in water, which is commonly used for the treatment of pain in the terminally ill.

Emulsions Colloidal suspensions of one liquid in another, usually an oil or fat and water. Examples: cod-liver oil, liquid paraffin.

Eye-drops Sterile preparations for instillation into the eye. Examples: cocaine, antibiotics, atropine, pilocarpine.

Eye lotions   Usually dispensed with instructions to dilute with an equal quantity of warm water to form a lotion isotonic with the lacrimal secretion and therefore non-irritating. Examples: boric acid, zinc sulphate compound.

Glycerins   Drugs for local application made up in glycerin. Examples: glycerin and ichthammol.

Inhalations   Preparations, commonly made up with industrial alcohol, of drugs to be added to hot water from which the patient inhales vapour. Examples: menthol, benzoin.

Irrigations   Solutions, commonly antiseptic or astringent, to be diluted with warm water for application to a cavity such as the vagina or the bladder. Examples: chlorhexidine (Hibitane) 1 in 5000, normal saline.

Linctuses   Preparations of drugs made up with a syrup base and flavouring agents, used as cough sedative and intended to be sipped from a spoon. Example: codeine linctus.

Liniments   Oily preparations, to be applied externally and locally. Example: methyl salicylate.

Mixtures   Liquid preparations of drugs in water, usually containing a number of ingredients. Examples: magnesium trisilicate, kaolin.

Nasal sprays   Water solutions of drugs to be applied to the nasal cavity with an atomizer. Examples: adrenaline, amethocaine. These are often made up locally on the instruction of a consultant.

Nebulizers These are packs of variable design but all employ the principle of delivering a single dose of a specific drug using either a trigger-release or finger pressure. The drug is inhaled orally or intra-nasally as a fine mist powder. Nebulizers may also be attached to oxygen therapy, when the drugs are initially filtered through water before being inhaled. Examples: ephedrine, salbutamol, sodium cromoglycate, which are used to relieve allergy, asthma or acute bronchitic attacks.

Ointments Drugs mixed with fatty substances, such as lanolin or soft paraffin, for external application. Examples: hydrocortisone, resorcinol.

Paints Fluid preparations, often of a slightly sticky nature, to be applied locally. Examples: iodine compound (Mandl's paint).

Pessaries Solid preparations, usually with a glycerin base, containing drugs intended to act locally in the vagina. Example: nystatin.

Pills Solid preparations of drugs formed into small balls and often sugar-coated. Example: digitoxin.

Poultices Drugs incorporated in a soft paste to be warmed and spread on a flannel or cotton backing and applied locally. Example: kaolin.

Powders Preparations of drugs in powder form to be mixed with, or swallowed with, water. Examples: compound effervescent (Seidlitz powder), magnesium trisilicate.

Sprays Drugs incorporated into a pressurized pack to

produce very fine droplets. Examples: Op-Site, Nobe-cutane.

Suppositories   Preparations of drugs incorporated in a cocoa butter or glycerin base for insertion into the rectum. Examples: glycerin, aminophylline.

Tablets   Preparations of drugs powdered and compressed. Examples: acetylsalicylic acid (aspirin), buto-barbitone (Soneryl).

12
Factors affecting the
Dosage of Drugs

The dosage of a drug is modified by certain conditions such as:

Age Young children can tolerate relatively large doses of some drugs, but react strongly to very small doses of others, notably opium preparations and barbiturates. Dosage for infants and children is usually calculated on the basis of the body weight, or on a percentage basis related to age. Barbiturates may give rise to confusion in some elderly patients, particularly those over 65.

Diet See monoamine oxidase inhibitors (p. 84).

Disease The action of any drug may be modified by the presence of disease. For example, in renal and liver failure, drugs are excreted at a slower rate than normal and therefore smaller doses may be given.

Cumulative action Certain drugs, if taken continually for any length of time, tend to accumulate in the body and may produce harmful effects, e.g. digitalis and large doses of chlorpromazine (Largactil).

Idiosyncrasy Some persons show symptoms of poisoning when given minute doses of certain drugs, e.g. iodine, iron dextran (Imferon), bromides. Even applications of lotions such as iodine or turpentine may produce toxic symptoms.

Tolerance The opposite of idiosyncrasy, for an individual may tolerate much larger doses than a normal person. Tolerance can be natural, or acquired by prolonged use of a drug such as opium, alcohol or arsenic.

Sensitivity reaction   A dramatic response to a drug, such as vomiting or development of a rash. Often associated with administration of serum or penicillin, particularly in patients with a history of asthma.

Habit   Persons who are habitually under the influence of a drug may require larger doses than is usual, e.g. opium.

Method of administration   Hypodermic and intra-muscular doses are usually smaller and rectal doses larger, than the dose of the same drug given by mouth. Intravenous administration is the fastest route for absorption of a drug.

13
Abbreviations in Prescriptions

Latin abbreviations are gradually being replaced by English versions which are considered safer. As the nurse may still meet Latin, a selective list is given below.

Abbreviation	Latin	English
aa	ana	of each (i.e. equal parts)
a.c.	ante cibum	before food
ad lib.	ad libitum	as much as desired
aq.	aqua	water
b.i.d./b.d.	bis in die	twice daily
c.	cum	with
dil.	dilutus	diluted
fl.	fluidium	fluid
o.m.	omne mane	every morning
o.n.	omne nocte	every night
p.c.	post cibum	after food
p.r.n.	pro re nata	as occasion arises (repeat when required)
q.d./q.i.d.	quater in die	four times daily
s.o.s.	si opus sit	if the occasion arises (a single dose)
stat.	statim	immediately
t.d./t.i.d.	ter in die	thrice daily
t.d.s.	ter die sumendus	to be taken three times a day

14
Vaccination and Immunization

Table V is an example of an immunization programme offered by the Health Authorities for children in the United Kingdom. Immunization is also offered to those individuals at risk from influenza and rabies and is available for people travelling to geographical areas where they may encounter the following diseases: yellow fever, cholera, typhoid and paratyphoid fever, and rickettsial infections. Travellers should always check with their travel agents on the current regulations or recommendations in force for particular countries at any given time.

Table V. A typical immunization programme

Vaccine	Minimum age	Comment
Tuberculin sensitivity test	Birth *or* 6 weeks *or* 12 years	Followed by BCG vaccination if required
Oral poliomyelitis		
1st dose	6 months	
2nd dose	8 months	
3rd dose	14 months	
Triple antigen (diphtheria + pertussis + tetanus toxoid)	Same time as polio	Pertussis in dispute but recommended
Measles	17 months	
Diphtheria, tetanus toxoid, polio	4½ years	Booster dose
Rubella	11 years	Girls only
Tetanus toxoid, polio	15 years	Booster dose
Hepatitis immunoglobulin	—	Available if at risk from hepatitis B infection
Smallpox	—	Not recommended as routine procedure, except in suspected smallpox areas

N.B. The ages quoted are guidelines only.

15
Chemotherapeutic and Antibiotic Agents

Chemotherapeutic drugs, which include the antibiotics, are a class of chemical substances which combat pathogenic organisms in the living tissue of the host. The action of the drug may be bacteriostatic, i.e. preventing the multiplication of bacteria and so enabling the body's defences to combat the infection satisfactorily, or bactericidal, i.e. lethal to invading organisms. Most chemotherapeutic agents are selective in action, being effective against certain organisms but not all; one factor in successful treatment, therefore, is the choice of drug.

Penicillin

The first and still one of the most widely used of the antibiotics is penicillin, produced from the mould *Pencillium notatum.*

Penicillin is effective against a number of common organisms including streptococci, staphylococci, pneumococci and gonococci. It is free from toxic side-effects and can be given in very large doses, but some people develop a sensitivity which is manifested by allergic reactions such as urticaria and even anaphylactic shock. For this reason patients should be asked if they have had previous penicillin treatment, and it may be necessary to give them a small test dose. One other important disadvantage of penicillin is the development of resistant strains of bacteria, particularly, *Staphylococcus aureus,* which produce an enzyme, penicillinase, which inactivates penicillin. Five main forms of penicillin are in general use:

1. *Benzylpenicillin (Penicillin G)*, a crystalline, soluble

form which is quickly absorbed into the blood stream when given by intramuscular injection. *Dosage* is of the order of 0.5–1g 4-hourly.

2. *Procaine penicillin* is slowly absorbed and therefore the effect is more prolonged than that of penicillin G. *Dosage:* 0.5–1 g twice daily by intramuscular injection.

3. *Phenoxymethylpenicillin (Penicillin V)* and *phenethicillin (Broxil)* are unaffected by the acid gastric juice and can therefore be given by mouth. *Dosage:* Penicillin V, 60–300 mg by mouth 4–6-hourly; Broxil, 150–250 mg by mouth, 4–6-hourly.

4. *Ampicillin* is an important broad spectrum penicillin and may be given by injection or orally.

5. *Cloxacillin* is not inactivated by penicillinases, and may be given by injection or orally. *Dosage:* 1.5–3g daily in divided doses.

Substances which hinder the excretion of penicillin and therefore help to maintain the level of the drug in the blood, such as probenicid (Benemid), may be given with penicillin.

Penicillin is now seldom used topically (although it may be employed in extensive burns) as this is particularly liable to produce sensitivity to the drug.

Streptomycin

Streptomycin is derived from another mould, *Streptomyces griseus.* Its main use is in the treatment of all forms of tuberculosis. *Dosage* = 0.5–0.75 g daily. Resistant strains of *Mycobacterium tuberculosis* are, however, readily produced; the combination of streptomycin with PAS and isoniazid (see p. 101) markedly reduces this tendency. Cycloserine and capreomycin are two alternative antibiotics which may be given if drug resistance to streptomycin develops.

Tetracyclines

A group of antibiotics, derived from varieties of *Streptomyces,* known as 'broad spectrum' antibiotics since they are effective against a wide range of bacteria, a few viruses and the Rickettsiae which cause typhus fever. They are liable to produce some uncomfortable side-effects such as a sore tongue, fungal infection of the mouth and diarrhoea; to combat these a vitamin B preparation is often administered at the same time. The four varieties of tetracycline are:

1. Chlortetracycline. ⎤ *Dosage:*
2. Tetracycline.   ⎬ 250 mg 4-hourly
3. Oxytetracycline.   ⎦ by mouth.
4. Demethylchlortetracycline. *Dosage:* 300 mg twice daily.

Chloramphenicol

This drug was originally derived from a form of *Streptomyces* but is now prepared synthetically. Its chief uses are in the treatment of typhoid fever and meningitis. It is effective against a number of organisms but has the disadvantage of depressing the formation of white blood cells if given in large doses, and for this reason its use has been restricted.

Erythromycin

This is the most active and most widely used of a group of antibiotics all derived from a type of *Streptomyces*. Erythromycin has a particular use in staphylococcal infections which have proved resistant to penicillin, although resistant strains to this drug can also be produced. *Dosage:* 200–500 mg 6-hourly, by mouth.

Polymyxins

A group of antibiotics obtained from cultures of *Bacillus polymyxa*. Polymyxin B is effective against infection with *Pseudomonas aeruginosa,* but has the disadvantage of exerting a toxic effect on the kidneys. It is not absorbed by the gut, so must be given intravenously or intramuscularly. *Dosage:* 60 mg 4-hourly by intramuscular injection. In cases of *Pseudomonas aeruginosa* meningitis the drug is given intrathecally, 5–10 mg in 1 ml of isotonic saline solution.

Nystatin

Also derived from *Streptomyces,* nystatin is used as a local application for fungal infections of the skin and mucous membranes.

Griseofulvin

This is obtained from a variety of penicillium mould and is effective against fungal infections of skin, hair and nails. *Dosage:* 250 mg 6-hourly, by mouth.

Cephalosporins

This group of antibiotics is similar in its action to the penicillin group and can be used as an alternative in 90% of those sensitive to pencillin. Cephalosporins have a broad spectrum of activity similar to that of ampicillin and can be given orally.

Non-absorbable Antibiotics

Under this classification are grouped a number of antibiotics which are either not absorbed or only slightly absorbed from the alimentary tract when given by mouth. Examples of these are neomycin and colistin. They are prescribed in the treatment of certain intestinal infections, such as bacillary dysentery, and prior to operations on the intestines, in order to reduce the number of intestinal micro-organisms.

Sulphonamides

The sulphonamides are of value in the treatment of a wide range of infections. They are especially valuable for urinary tract infections involving gram-negative bacteria, for reducing intestinal bacteria before surgery, and in the treatment of meningococcal meningitis. Examples of sulphonamide compounds in general use are:

1. *Sulphadimidine,* which is effective against a wide variety of infections, including those due to streptococci, pneumococci and meningococci. Since it has a low toxicity it is one of the most generally useful of the sulphonamide compounds. *Dosage:* initial dose 3–4 g, then 1.0–1.5 g 6-hourly by injection.

2. *Sulphadiazine,* which is particularly useful in the treatment of meningococcal meningitis as it is absorbed into the cerebrospinal fluid. *Dosage:* initial dose 3–4 g, then 1.0–1.5 g 4-hourly by injection.

3. *Phthalylsulphathiazole*, which is used in the treatment of intestinal infections as it is only slowly absorbed from the alimentary tract. *Dosage:* 2–12 g daily in divided doses.

4. *Sulphamethizole,* which is used for treatment of urinary infections. *Dosage:* 1 g daily in divided doses.

5. *Sulphadimethoxine*, which is a long-acting sulphonamide. *Dosage:* initial dose 1–2 g, then 500 mg daily.

6. *Sulphacetamide*, which is used for local applications, for example as eye drops in the treatment of conjunctivitis.

Sulphone Compounds

These are related to the sulphonamides and are used in the treatment of leprosy. The most widely used is dapsone. Dapsone solution for injection is prepared in the strength of 0.25 g per ml. Dapsone is also dispensed in 100 mg tablets. The dose is prescribed in accordance with the needs of the patient and up to 400 mg may be given twice weekly.

Antituberculosis Drugs

Ethambutol This drug has a similar action to isoniazid and may be used in its place in combination with streptomycin. *Dosage:* 300–400 mg daily by mouth.

Isoniazid (INAH) This preparation has an effective action against *Mycobacterium tuberculosis*, but if it is used alone drug resistance can develop quickly. For this reason isoniazid is always used in combination, usually with streptomycin. *Dosage:* 100–300 mg daily by mouth.

Rifampicin This drug interferes with bacterial metabolism and its main use is in the treatment of tuberculosis. It is prescribed in combination with isoniazid orally as tablets or syrups.

Pyrazinamide This drug is used as an adjunct to other antituberculosis drugs.

Para-aminosalicylic acid (PAS) This drug is only weakly effective against *Mycobacterium tuberculosis*, but used in conjunction with other antituberculosis drugs it helps to prevent the development of drug-resistant strains of the organism. It is used as a last line of treatment. *Dosage:* 12–20 g daily by mouth.

Streptomycin See p. 97.

The administration of antituberculosis drugs may be continued for periods of up to 2 years.

Nitrofurans

This group of drugs is effective against a wide range of both gram-positive and gram-negative bacteria, including *Staphylococcus aureus*. They are useful in the treatment of infections where the organism has developed resistance to other chemotherapeutic agents. Examples of this group are nitrofurantoin which is excreted in the urine and therefore effective in the treatment of urinary infections (*dosage:* 100 mg by mouth 6-hourly) and nitrofurazone which is used as a local application for wounds and skin conditions.

16
Hormones and Hormone-like Agents

Thyroid Gland Hormones

The thyroid gland manufactures an iodine-containing hormone known as *thyroxine* which profoundly affects the metabolic processes which convert food substances into energy and new tissue cells. In childhood it is one of the main factors controlling growth and development. Thyroxine is therefore used in the medical treatment of hypothyroidism (reduced thyroid activity), which may be congenital (cretinism) or develop in adult life (myxoedema). Preparations available at present include thyroxine and liothyronine.

Thyroxine Tablets

These tablets contain pure L-thyroxine sodium. In the elderly, or those with heart disease or hypertension, the drug is introduced at very low dosage and increased on a sliding scale over a period of four to six weeks. A cretinous baby may be prescribed a dose of 0.025 mg daily and the dose increased by 0.025 mg fortnightly, until the optimum dose is reached, just below that which causes diarrhoea.

Liothyronine Tablets

Liothyronine is a fast-acting and effective thyroid hormone, a single dose giving maximum effect within 24 hours. It is used exclusively for myxoedema coma and psychosis, both rare conditions. This drug is usually combined with hydrocortisone since the adrenocortical function is usually depressed in prolonged hypothyroidism. Liothyronine may also be used to establish the diagnosis in doubtful cases of hyperthyroidism.

Undesirable effects of thyroxine-based drugs are those which parallel hyperthyroidism. Angina pectoris or heart failure may be induced with high doses. In the elderly, atrial fibrillation can be caused with only a slight overdose.

Calcitonin is also secreted by the thyroid gland and may be given by injection to treat cases of increased calcium in the blood (hypercalcaemia).

Antithyroid Drugs and Radioiodine

In hyperthyroidism (increased thyroid activity) various preparations may be used to suppress the production of excess thyroxine. These are listed below. (See also p. 82.)

Iodine

Iodine diminishes the blood supply to the thyroid gland and temporarily controls hyperthyroidism. Its chief use is as a preoperative treatment, given for 10 to 14 days prior to thyroidectomy. Preparations available include:

Potassium iodide: 30–120 mg daily in divided doses.
Aqueous iodine solution (Lugol's Solution) consisting of iodine 5% plus potassium iodide 10%: 0.3–1 ml daily in divided doses.

Thiourea Derivatives

These act by blocking the incorporation of iodine into the organic precursors of thyroid hormone so that less thyroxine is produced. Preparations available include:

Propylthiouracil: 200 mg daily for eight weeks followed by a maintenance dose of 50 mg.

Carbimazole (Neo-Mercazole): 40 mg daily until symptoms subside then 5 mg daily.

The patient should show improvement within about a week, measured in terms of emotional state, weight gain and slower pulse rate, and should achieve a normal thyroid state within about eight weeks. A pregnant woman should receive the smallest possible dose if she is suffering from hyperthyroidism and the lactating mother should not be given antithyroid drugs as they are concentrated in the breast milk. Blood disorders may occur in the first two months of treatment with the thiourea derivatives.

Potassium Perchlorate

This is an alternative drug used in those patients who are allergic to thiourea derivatives which also blocks the synthesis of thyroid hormone.

Radioiodine (^{131}I and ^{132}I)

These radioactive substances taken orally can be used to measure the activity of the thyroid gland, or in higher doses to treat selected cases of hyperthyroidism, usually in the elderly. See p. 137.

Parathyroid Hormone

The parathyroid glands, situated on the posterior aspect of the thyroid gland, secrete parathyroid hormone (parathormone), which contributes to the control of the metabolism and blood level of calcium in the body. Hyperparathyroidism (over-secretion of parathyroid hormone), is generally associated with the presence of a tumour, and is treated by removal of the tumour. Hypoparathyroidism (under-secretion of parathyroid hormone) may occur following thyroidectomy, and may result in tetany due to a decreased level of calcium in the blood. The treatment is to give calcium, orally or by intravenous injection (calcium gluconate injection 10% solution at the rate of 2 ml per minute).

Adrenal Gland Hormones

Cortical Hormones

The cortex of the adrenal gland produces three differing types of hormone classified as follows:

1. *Mineralocorticoids (e.g. aldosterone),* which are concerned with the regulation of electrolytes and influences the retention of salt and water, and the excretion of potassium.

2. *Glucocorticoids (e.g. hydrocortisone),* which are concerned with the metabolism of proteins and carbohydrates, and the conversion and storage of glycogen.

3. *Androgens (e.g. testosterone),* which are concerned with the building of proteins in the body and the development of the secondary sexual characteristics.

Natural or synthesized forms of these hormones, also known as steroids, can be used in replacement therapy, immunosuppression therapy, to suppress chronic inflammation, and also in diagnostic testing.

If these drugs are given over long periods, side effects are likely to occur, such as salt and water retention leading to oedema, loss of potassium, hypertension, changes in appearance (the so called 'moon face' or 'orange stick man'), mental disturbances and peptic ulceration. The administration of cortical hormones suppresses the normal activity of the adrenal glands, and these drugs are therefore withdrawn gradually to prevent acute adrenal deficiency. Those patients on replacement therapy must never be without a constant and regular supply of their prescribed drug. Should the patient suffer an intercurrent illness or be involved in an emergency or accident, the dose of the drug will need to be increased, and the patient should be strongly advised to always carry a card stating his/her diagnosis, drug, and the prescribed dose.

Hydrocortisone (cortisol) is the principal naturally-occurring steroid. It can be given by all routes including intra-articularly. *Hydrocortisone succinate* and *hydrocortisone acetate* are the two most commonly used compounds and can be given for immediate or prolonged effect.

Cortisone is converted to hydrocortisone by the liver; it cannot therefore be given for topical application and has a very limited use in patients with liver disease. It is used mainly as replacement therapy.

Prednisone and *prednisolone* are both predominantly anti-inflammatory. They are five times more effective than naturally occurring steroids, and can thus be given in smaller doses. They are sometimes used in the palliative treatment of malignant disease.

Methylprednisolone is similar to prednisolone.

Triamcinalone has virtually no sodium-retaining effect, but may cause muscle-wasting, and anorexia and mental depression at high doses.

Dexamethasone and *betamethasone* are similar

steroids with effective anti-inflammatory properties.

Fludrocortisone is a synthetic preparation with similar properties to aldosterone. It is used in combination with cortisone in the treatment of Addison's disease and following bilateral adrenalectomy, to prevent excessive loss of sodium.

Aldosterone is the naturally-occurring salt-retaining cortical hormone. It has limited application in therapy, since fludrocortisone is equally effective and is not inactivated when taken orally.

Medullary Hormones

The medulla of the adrenal gland produce hormones which have effects similar to those produced by stimulation of the sympathetic nervous system, i.e. increased heart rate, raised blood pressure, and the release of glycogen as fuel for immediate use. In medical practice these substances are used to relieve bronchial spasm in asthma and to counteract anaphylactic reactions.

Adrenaline (epinephrine) is the main hormone of the adrenal medulla and is used in the treatment of asthmatic attacks, allergic conditions and anaphylaxis. It can be used locally to control bleeding and can be combined with local anaesthetics to slow down their absorption into the body.

Ephedrine is chemically similar to adrenaline but with a longer-acting effect. It is used as a bronchodilator, in heart block, as a mydriatic, and as a mucosal vasoconstrictor. Its side-effects are those of a stimulant to the central nervous system; insomnia, alertness, anxiety, tremor and nausea.

Isoprenaline (isoproterenol) is a derivative of adrenaline which relaxes bronchial spasm and blood vessels and is also a vigorous stimulant to the heart. It is given as sublingual tablets or orally (Saventrine) for slow release. For asthma an aerosol spray 1% is preferred, being more effective than the sublingual tablets; the benefit of the spray is felt within 30 seconds.

Other drugs which produce a broncho-dilatory action are:

Orciprenaline (Alupent) orally, by inhalation or by aerosol spray.

Salbutamol (Ventolin) orally, by inhalation or by aerosol spray.

Isoetharine (Numotac) prepared as a slow-release tablet.

Terbutaline (Bricanyl) orally, by injection or by aerosol spray.

Pituitary Gland Hormones

The anterior lobe of the pituitary gland secretes growth hormone, gonadotrophins (FSH and LH), corticotrophin (ACTH), thyroid stimulating hormone (TSH) and prolactin. The posterior lobe secretes vasopressin (ADH) and oxytocin.

Growth hormone is available from human pituitaries but is only prescribed in diagnostically certain cases of pituitary deficiency.

Gonadotrophins are obtained from both man and animal sources although animal sources are not very satisfactory. Human gonadotrophin is obtained from the urine of pregnant women, and can induce ovulation in some types of infertility.

Corticotrophin (ACTH) stimulates the activity of the cortex of the adrenal gland. It is a short-acting hormone and its use has been superseded by hydrocortisone and its synthetic preparations.

Prolactin secretion can be stimulated by the administration of such drugs as the phenothiazines, tricyclic antidepressants, reserpine, and methyldopa.

Vasopressin (Pitressin) is also known as the antidiuretic hormone (ADH). It is used in hypothalamic or pituitary diabetes insipidus, and to reduce portal venous pressure in those patients with hepatic cirrhosis. The drug can be given as a spray, snuff, or by injection.

Oxytocin (Syntocinon) stimulates contraction of the uterus and is used in obstetric practice for this purpose. The hormone is usually given by the intravenous route. Oxytocin may be combined with prostaglandins for the induction of labour. In the past oxytocin was also used in the treatment of post partum haemorrhage but has now, by and large, been replaced by *ergometrine*.

Sex Hormones

The natural male androgen is *testosterone*, which is mainly secreted by the interstitial cells of the testes and is necessary for the development of secondary sexual characteristics and normal spermatogenesis. The androgens also increase protein metabolism and during adolescence a great amount of new protein is laid down as muscle; this acounts for the greater muscle mass in males.

Oestrone and *oestradiol* are the naturally-occurring female hormones. These oestrogens are responsible for the development of the female genital tract, and the breasts and other secondary sexual characteristics. The oestrogens are also necessary for normal pregnancy and the accompanying enlargement of the breasts.

Testosterone can be used therapeutically in testicular deficiency and in carcinoma of the breast in the female. It is also used for its anabolic effect to increase weight in senile osteoporosis and in debilitating diseases. Examples of testosterone preparations include:

Methyltestosterone, given as sublingual tablets.

Testosterone propionate, given intramuscularly.

Testosterone enanthate, given intramuscularly, which has a long lasting effect.

The virilizing effects of testosterone when used in the female patient can be overcome by the use of synthetic androgens known as anabolic steroids, e.g. *nandrolone.*

Oestrogens are used as a replacement therapy in hypo-ovarian conditions, in the treatment of hormone-dependent malignancy of the prostate gland, and in cancer of the breast in post-menopausal women. Preparations include:

Oestradiol, the natural oestrogen, given intramuscularly two or three times weekly.

Oestrone sulphate has fewer toxic effects than other oral oestrogens.

Ethinyloestradiol is a very potent semi-synthetic oestrogen.

Stilboestrol was the first synthetic oestrogen and is often prescribed to males in the treatment of cancer of the prostate gland.

Dienoestrol and *hexoestrol* are similar to stilboestrol.

The Contraceptive Pill

The contraceptive pill is used to prevent pregnancy by inhibiting ovulation. It inhibits the hypothalamus thereby preventing the pituitary from releasing gonadotrophins. It also alters the endometrium so that

implantation is less likely to occur. Oral contraceptives
fall into three groups:

1. Oestrogen and progestagen as a combined preparation which is begun on the fifth day after menstruation and continued for 21 days, followed by a
   7-day interval.
2. Oestrogen and progestagen taken sequentially,
   oestrogen taken alone for 15–21 days, then accompanied by progestagen on the last five to ten days
   of the course.
3. Progestagen alone. This method is less reliable
   than the above two, relying mainly on its action on
   the cervical mucus, for its contraceptive effect.

There are recognized risks in taking the pill, one of the
important ones being the risk of deep vein thrombosis.
This is especially important in those patients who may
require surgery, and for this reason the pill should be
stopped for some time prior to hospitalization.

Pancreatic Hormones

The pancreas secretes insulin from the beta cells and
glucagon from the alpha cells of the Islets of
Langerhans. Both hormones are used in the treatment
of diabetes mellitus. Preparations of insulin are available in both quick- and long-acting varieties. After
diagnosis and stabilization, diabetic patients follow one
of three possible regimens:

1. Insulin and diet.
2. Oral hypoglycaemic tablets and diet.
3. Diet alone.

These patients require re-evaluation of their diabetes
at regular intervals, as well as prior to surgery and
during any intercurrent illness. Regardless of their
normal regimen, insulin may, at times, be required to
keep their condition stable.

Insulin Preparations

1. *Soluble insulin,* a quick-acting preparation which is easy to administer subcutaneously. It is often used to stabilize those diabetics in need of insulin and is always used in the treatment of diabetic ketoacidosis. The major disadvantage is the frequency of injections required.

2. *Insulin zinc suspension (IZS),* whose period of action may be short (Semilente), intermediate (Lente) or long (Ultralente).

3. *Protamine zinc insulin (PZI),* a very long-acting insulin which is similar to Ultralente. It may be prescribed in combination with soluble insulin, in which case the soluble insulin should be drawn into the syringe first.

4. *Isophane insulin,* an intermediate-acting preparation, which can be combined with soluble insulin.

Occasionally a patient is allergic to insulin of bovine origin and the purer form which comes from the pancreas of the pig (porcine) is prescribed. Insulin should be stored in a thermostatically controlled refrigerator, otherwise changes may occur in the insulin, causing reactions within the patient.

Preparations of insulin will continue for some time to be issued in single, double and quadruple strengths although these latter strengths will eventually be replaced by 100 unit (U100) strength insulin. This relatively new insulin has been recently introduced as part of an international effort to standardize strengths and thus reduce errors. Insulin should only be drawn up in an insulin syringe as any other type of syringe will lead to error. For long term use, the patient should be issued with a glass syringe; for temporary use, such as in hospital, disposable types of syringe are available.

The standard insulin syringe is designed for use with single strength insulin and is calibrated either in 50 or 100 units (marks). However, since insulin may be supplied in various strengths, when calculating the numbers of marks needed the nurse should:

> Divide by 1 when using single strength (20 unit/ml).
> Divide by 2 when using double strength (40 unit/ml).
> Divide by 4 when using quadruple strength (80 unit/ml).
> Use only a 100 unit syringe when using 100 unit (U100) strength – the number of units can then be read directly off the syringe.

For example if 32 units of soluble insulin were prescribed then the patient would need:

> 32 marks of single strength.
> 16 marks of double strength.
> 8 marks of quadruple strength.
> 32 units, read directly off the syringe, of 100 strength.

Glucagon

Glucagon mobilizes glycogen from the liver but this physiological source of glucose is quickly exhausted. Glucagon is used in the early phase of hypoglycaemia when intravenous glucose is not readily available, and for this reason may be prescribed for unstable diabetics at home. Its maximum effective time is only 45 minutes and hospital treatment is essential within 15 minutes of the second injection.

Oral Hypoglycaemic Agents

Oral hypoglycaemic agents are commonly used in preference to insulin in those patients who have partially secreting insulin cells. These oral compounds are either derived from the sulphonamides (sulphonylureas) or the guanides (biguanides). The sulphonylureas promote the activity of partially-secreting insulin cells, the biguanides reduce the absorption of carbohydrate from the gut and increase the uptake of insulin in the peripheral tissues, providing insulin is present.

Sulphonylureas *Tolbutamide (Rastinon)* is rapidly excreted and two to three doses are required daily. *Chlorpropamide (Diabinese)* is slowly excreted, and only one dose is necessary per day. *Acetohexamide, tolazamide* and *glibenclamide* are alternative sulphonylureas which, unlike tolbutamide and chlorpropamide, allow the patient to take alcohol.

Biguanides *Metformin (Glucophage)* is prescribed singly or in combination with a sulphonylurea for those who are insulin-independent and also obese, for example, those with maturity onset diabetes. This drug may cause malabsorption of vitamin B12 from the gut.

17
Chemical Disinfectants and Antiseptics in Common Use

Many substances which are named as disinfectants are not necessarily bactericidal to all living organisms. For disinfectants to be effective in sterilizing equipment, they must be used at the prescribed strength for a specific period of time and must be in direct contact with the article to be sterilized, which must have been adequately cleansed and rinsed before disinfection. Unless these principles are applied, chemical disinfection may well prove unreliable. Where any doubt exists, the advice of the bacteriologist or cross-infection control officer should be sought.

It is standard practice in hospitals for the pharmacy department to label stock bottles of antiseptics and disinfectants with the solution strength and the purpose for which the solution is to be used. The nurse should adhere strictly to these instructions as a lotion used in either too weak or too strong a solution may be potentially harmful to the patient, to the nurse or to the equipment. For example, chlorhexidine (Hibitane) is used in different strengths and may be in either aqueous or alcoholic solution, depending on its application. Table VI gives some examples of commonly used disinfectants and antiseptics.

To avoid painful smarting, spirit-based antiseptics should not come into contact with the skin directly after it has been shaved, or with mucous membranes. Iodine in spirit may cause blistering if it is not allowed to evaporate after application to the skin.

The problems of disinfection have been greatly reduced over the years with the increased use of disposable equipment; wherever practicable and safe such items should be introduced since they reduce the risks of cross-infection. Examples of equipment available in disposable form include linen, crockery, cutlery, dressing packs, catheters, syringes, nail brushes, shaving equipment, sputum containers, and a wide variety of instruments. Such equipment is used once only, then incinerated.

Linen should not be disinfected on the wards. Infected or foul linen should be sealed in an impermeable bag, placed in a second bag and clearly labelled 'infected' before being sent to the laundry. Many hospitals use coloured laundry bags for this purpose.

Fumigation of rooms is usually reserved for cases of anthrax; if there is any doubt about whether fumigation is required the cross-infection officer should be contacted for advice.

Table VI. Some disinfectants and antiseptics and their uses

Chemical	Strength	Uses
Acridines A group of dyes including aminacrine, flavine, euflavine, and proflavine hemisulphate	1-in-1000	Aqueous solution: swabbing wounds Alcohol solution: skin antisepsis
Chlorine preparations Eusol Sodium hypochlorite	0·5–2% 1% 1-in-80 (Milton) 10%	Wound irrigation or dressing Disinfecting stainless steel bed cradles Disinfecting feeding bottles and teats Disinfecting baths or sinks Soaking polypropylene urinals Disinfecting bedpans containing viral faecal infections

Chlorhexidine	0·0075% aqueous solution (Hibitane)	Adding to humidifying tanks of incubators
	20% (Hibiscrub)	Reducing bacterial flora on hands Skin antisepsis
Chlorhexidine + cetrimide (in sachets)	0·5% in 70% alcohol	Skin antisepsis
	0·05% and 0·5%	Skin antisepsis
	0·0075% and 0·075%	Swabbing plastic, rubber or varnished surfaces
Chlorhexidine + sodium nitrate	0·02% and 0·1%	Instrument storage (rendered sterile within 30 minutes)
Chlorhexidine + isopropyl alcohol (in sachets)	0·5% and 70%	Skin antisepsis before injection, venepuncture or deep needling procedures
		Wiping rubber- or plastic-capped ampoules
Glutaraldehyde (Cidex)	2%	Storage of instruments (solution effective for 7 days)
		Sterilization of endoscopic and cystoscopic instruments (immerse for 3 hours)
Hydrogen peroxide	2·5–20 volumes of available oxygen; diluted as required	Cleansing wounds and cavities such as the mouth

Chemical	Strength	Uses
Iodine	0·75% (povidone-iodine)	Skin antisepsis before surgery
		Compress for contaminated wounds
	1–2·5% in 70% alcohol	Skin antisepsis
Phenolic solution (Stericol)	2%	Disinfecting stainless steel basins
		Disinfecting walls, floors, ceilings in specific risk areas, e.g. theatre
	1%	Immersing soiled instruments immediately after use (suction jars filled to one-tenth capacity)
White disinfectant	1-in-160	Covering contents of bedpans of known and suspected infection with *Salmonella*, *Shigella* or staphylococcal enteritis for 30 minutes before discarding
	1-in-640	Disinfecting unvarnished surfaces

18
X-ray Examinations

X-ray examination interpretation is based on shadows, and pathology is recognized by either addition to or subtraction from these shadows. It is therefore essential to eliminate from the field of investigation any substances likely to cast additional shadows on the radiograph. Such extraneous substances include:

Clothing (silk and artificial silk, buttons, elastic, pins, hair-clips).

Radio-opaque dressings or applications, e.g. those impregnated with iodine, lead lotion or kaolin.

Elastoplast.

Kaolin, Thermogene wool.

Rubber tubes.

Wigs, breast prostheses, dentures, artificial eyes.

Metallic splints (except aluminium).

Plaster of Paris splints (these obscure detail, particularly while still wet, but a reasonable radiograph of fractures through dry plaster of Paris is possible).

Bowel content and gas cast shadows and obscure detail, which make pathology of the urinary system, coccyx and even lumbar spine difficult to recognize.

Adherence to recognized rules in the preparation of the patient aids the accuracy of the subsequent diagnosis, saves the patient the inconvenience and possible discomfort of a repeated examination, and saves time, labour and cost in the radiography department. *If there is any doubt as to the correct procedure in any case, specific instructions should be sought from the radiologist.* The patient should receive a reasonable explanation of what is involved in the examination and be told that he/she may need to spend some considerable time in the radiography department. Nurses should ensure that patients are both warm and comfortable before leaving the ward. Elderly, confused, unconscious or infant patients should always be escorted to and from the radiography department, and the nurse should, if possible, remain with the patient during the X-ray procedure. Many hospitals now have television cameras and monitor screens linked to the screening unit and the room need not be so dark as formerly.

The Alimentary System

Barium Meal Examination

The contrast medium used for this examination is barium sulphate. Various proprietary preparations are also used.

The object of the preparation procedure is to have the patient's stomach empty at the time when the examination is made. No food or drink is allowed for at least six hours prior to the barium meal, and many radiologists prefer 12 hours' starvation. No aperient should be given within 24 hours of the examination and any medicine containing heavy metals, e.g. bismuth, should be discontinued for at least two days previously. The examination takes between 24 and 48 hours; no food is usually allowed until the stomach is seen to be empty and no aperients or enemas are permitted until the examination is complete. It is helpful if the patient is able to stand during the examination, so if he has been confined to bed for some time, he should be allowed to sit out of bed and to stand for a day or two before the visit to the radiography department.

A 'follow-through' examination may be required; in this case the patient may have his prescribed diet after the first examination but no aperient may be given until the whole examination is completed.

Barium Enema Examination

The object of the preparation of the patient is to clear the colon of faeces and gas. An aperient is given on the day before the examination and a bisacodyl (Dulcolax) suppository or rectal washout is given just prior to the barium enema. Where possible the patient should be encouraged to walk, or move in bed, to help in the expulsion of the flatus. A light diet is usually allowed on the day of the examination. A film may be required 24 hours after the enema and in this case no aperient or enema should be given until the whole examination is complete.

Gall-Bladder: Cholecystography

The object of the preparation is first to empty the gall-bladder in order that the dye may be concentrated in it, and then to encourage the dye-filled gall-bladder to empty before the final films are taken.

An aperient is given two days before the examination, the dose required depending on what suits the patient. On the evening prior to the examination, a light meal of non-fatty foods is taken: fresh vegetables cooked without fat, fruit or fruit juices, lean meat, toast or bread, coffee and tea are permitted. No fried or fatty foods, e.g. milk, butter, eggs or salad dressing, must be eaten, and apart from a small amount of water, the patient must have nothing else to eat or drink until after the X-ray examination. Smoking should also be avoided.

On the night before the examination, radio-opaque capsules are swallowed with a little water. The dose depends on the size and weight of the patient. The capsules render the gall-bladder opaque to the X-ray. It is important that the capsules are swallowed whole and not chewed. After the first films have been taken, a pre-packed fat-containing preparation is given before further films are taken. The instructions issued by the radiography department may differ from this routine, and in some instances where one dose fails to outline the gall-bladder, two doses may be required.

Biligrafin or Telepaque may also be used to outline the biliary tract. It should be noted that any of these preparations may produce side effects such as nausea, vomiting and diarrhoea in some patients; Biloptin is thought to produce the least side effects.

Endoscopic Retrograde Cholangiopancreatography (ERCP)

A fibroptic examination of the bile and pancreatic ducts combined with the use of contrast media. The patient is prepared by starving for 3–4 hours. A mild aperient is given to empty the lower bowel. Intravenous sedation such as diazepam is used and a local anaesthetic is given to dull the pharynx. A narrow bore cannula is inserted into the ducts via the ampulla of Vater which are then filled with contrast media. Serial X-rays are taken while the duct is examined visually. This test can determine biliary lesions and pancreatic obstruction.

The Urinary Tract

Straight Radiograph of the Urinary Tract

This examination consists of taking films of the urinary tract without the use of contrast media.

Intravenous Pyelography

The object of the preparation is to have the bowel empty and to concentrate the urine.

On the *first day* of the preparation the patient is allowed a light diet but fluids are restricted. He should have an aperient in the evening — usually a vegetable laxative is ordered.

On the *second day* the same procedure is repeated.

On the *day of the examination* no fluids are allowed for at least six hours prior to the examination. A light breakfast is allowed. It is very important that the aperient given on the previous evening is effective and in order to prevent accumulation of gas in the intestine the patient should be encouraged to walk about if this is possible. The patient must empty the bladder immediately prior to the examination.

The contrast media used for this examination are iodine-containing solutions such as diodone (Uriodone), Conray and Hypaque. The radiologist should be warned in advance if the patient is sensitive to iodine. In some cases, where the blood urea level exceeds 6.6 mmol/litre, the doctor may decide to introduce the dye by intravenous drip as this gives a better concentration in the urinary tract; it is then not necessary to restrict fluids before the examination.

Retrograde or Instrumental Pyelography

This examination is carried out by injecting a contrast medium — a sterile solution of sodium iodide — into the pelvices of the kidneys by means of ureteric catheters. A cystoscope is passed first and the ureters are then catheterized. Usually about 7 ml of the solution is required to fill the pelvis of the kidney; the injection is stopped as soon as the patient complains of pain. The examination may be performed under general anaesthesia, when the patient will require routine preparation. On his return from the examination the ureteric catheters may still be in position; these should not be removed until the nurse is clearly instructed to do so.

Micturating Cystogram and Cysto-uretrogram

No specific preparation of the patient is required for this examination. A urinary catheter is passed, the bladder emptied, and contrast medium is injected through the catheter until the bladder is moderately full. The catheter is withdrawn and radiographs are taken while the patient is asked to 'strain' but to hold the urine, and then to pass urine into a receptacle provided. This examination may be used in the investigation of stress incontinence in women patients, of urinary infections in children, and to detect reflux of urine from the bladder along the ureters. It may also be done in males to detect urethral stricture.

The Lumbar Spine, Sacrum and Pelvis

In some cases no preparation of the patient is carried out prior to taking the films; in others the preparation described for radiography of the urinary tract may be ordered.

The Chest

Chest radiographs require no preparation, unless a bronchogram is to be carried out, beyond the removal of all clothing likely to cast shadows.

Bronchography

The contrast media used in this examination are iodized oils (Lipiodil and Dionosil). The medium may be introduced into the bronchi through a special syringe with a curved dropper attached which drops the oil into the trachea via the mouth. A local anaesthetic spray is required to anaesthetize the pharynx. An alternative method is to insert a short curved cannula into the trachea through the cricothyroid membrane. This may be carried out under a general anaesthetic.

Premedication may be ordered in the form of a sedative drug and an injection of atropine. The patient is not usually allowed any food within six hours of the examination, as there is a tendency to vomit.

After the examination it is important that the patient should not take any food or drink until the effects of the local anaesthetic have completely disappeared and the cough reflex is re-established. Postural drainage may be ordered before and after the examination.

Fallopian Tubes: Salpingography

Salpingography consists of taking films of the pelvis after the introduction of iodized oil into the uterine tubes. The oil is introduced through an intrauterine nozzle attached to a special syringe. The same preparation is required as for straight radiography of the urinary tract. This examination is not undertaken during menstruation. Premedication may be ordered.

The Brain

Cerebral Angiography

This is used to demonstrate the cerebral blood vessels by introducing a contrast medium into the carotid or vertebral arteries. The radiographs obtained may demonstrate such abnormalities as an aneurysm, a tumour of the brain or a haematoma resulting from a subdural or extradural haemorrhage; any one of these may displace an artery from its normal position.

With the patient under a local or general anaesthetic, the contrast medium is introduced into the carotid or vertebral artery through a length of plastic tubing using a special needle. Several films are then taken in different planes.

Encephalography

A lumbar puncture is carried out and a measured quantity of air, equal in volume to the cerebrospinal fluid removed, is injected into the sub-arachnoid space. This air, being lighter than the cerebrospinal fluid, then rises rapidly into the communicating ventricles of the brain. A series of films of the skull is then taken as in ventriculography (see below). The possibility of headache following this procedure is reduced if the patient is allowed to rest in the prone position and only one pillow is used for his head.

Ventriculography

Radiographs of the skull are taken after the injection of air into the ventricles of the brain. The procedure involves making trephine holes through the parietal bones, removing cerebrospinal fluid from the ventricles and injecting air. This operation is carried out by the surgeon in theatre and the usual preparations for any cranial operation are required. The appropriate area of the scalp must be shaved and the skin prepared. The usual reason for the examination is to aid in the diagnosis or location of a brain tumour, and the operation for removal of the tumour is performed at once if the radiography findings confirm the diagnosis.

This procedure may be followed by severe headache and/or nausea in the patient, who may require sedation on return to the ward and bedrest for several hours.

Myelography

Myelography is used to demonstrate any obstruction of the passage of cerebrospinal fluid down the spinal canal, such as tumour or disc protrusion. The procedure is similar to that for encephalography, using a contrast medium in place of air. If the suspected lesion is in the cervical region the injection is given via the cisterna magna as in cisternal puncture. If the lesion is thought to be in the lumber region, a water-soluble contrast media is injected to demonstrate not only the spinal canal but also the nerve roots. Films are taken with the patient sitting upright to avoid the contrast media rising above the second lumbar vertebra. Following the procedure it is important that the patient is kept in the semi-recumbent position for some time.

The Cardiovascular System

Arteriography

This is used to demonstrate the blood supply to a particular area. For example, in femoral arteriography an opaque medium, such as Hypaque, Urografin or Conray, is introduced via the femoral artery to demonstrate the blood supply to the lower limbs and the kidneys (renal arteriography). This procedure is not unusual in pregnancy.

The patient is prepared for a general anaesthetic, or a local anaesthetic may be used. The pubic area is shaved and the skin is cleansed. A thin plastic tube or catheter is introduced into the femoral artery with a special needle and passed along the artery to the required position. The contrast medium is then injected and the films taken. Alternatively, a narrow beam of radiation about 12mm in width is used to scan down the length of the artery, producing a series of films inside a long film holder called a cassette.

Following arteriography, observation of the site of the injection in the groin is important and should continue for several hours to avoid the complication of haemorrhage from the femoral artery.

Cardiac Catheterization (Cardio-angiography)

This may be used to detect congenital heart lesions and other types of heart disease. A long opaque catheter is introduced through one of the right arm veins into the right atrium, its course being watched on a television monitor screen. To demonstrate the left side of the heart the catheter is introduced via the femoral artery, as in arteriography. Before the contrast medium is injected, the cardiac catheter may be connected to a manometer to record pressures in the heart. Blood samples may be taken through it to assess the oxygen saturation in the various chambers of the heart and great vessels. For these investigations a local anaesthetic is used for adults, but a general anaesthetic may be required for a child.

Patients should be warned and reassured beforehand about the amount of complicated equipment which will face them on arrival in the radiography room.

Radioactive Isotopes

Other types of ray which may be used for therapy are those obtained from radioactive substances (radioisotopes), either in the form of sealed sources, such as radon seeds, or as unsealed sources in liquid form, such as radioactive iodine. Unsealed sources may also be used in diagnosis; they are given in small tracer quantities to a patient as a drink or injection, and the part under investigation is then scanned. The liver, brain, circulation and lungs may be investigated in this way (see p. 136).

Computerized Axial Tomography (Cat Scan)

This non-invasive X-ray technique of scanning soft body tissue can reveal unusual density or altered anatomical shape arising from, for example, a tumour. Films are taken in a series and build up a picture which can be retained in the computer's memory. These can then be referred to as often as is required to make a diagnosis, to suggest further investigations, or as the basis of a treatment plan. Minimal preparation of the patient is required apart from the general principles outlined at the beginning of this chapter.

19
The Therapeutic Use of X-rays and Radioactive Substances

X-rays and the radiations from both naturally-occurring radioactive elements, such as radium, and artificially produced radioactive isotopes of certain elements all have similar fundamental properties. They are all forms of energy propagated in wave form and are able to penetrate materials opaque to visible light. These radiations affect living cells and in sufficient quantities can destroy living tissue. The therapeutic use of radioactive substances is based on the fact that some cells are more readily damaged than others. Rapidly dividing and growing cells are more radio-sensitive than older cells, therefore the cells of a rapidly growing malignant tumour can be killed by a dose which, if carefully distributed, produces little permanent damage to the surrounding healthy tissues.

Deep X-ray Treatment

'Deep X-ray' implies the use of penetrating X-rays produced by the bombardment of a target by electrons travelling at high speed. The energy required for this is obtained using high voltage electricity, of the order of 180–100 000 kV or higher. This form of treatment is most frequently used in cases of malignant growth, either alone or in combination with surgery.

The majority of the patients require a large dose, spread over a period of several weeks, in order that a lethal dose can be delivered at the site of the growth without producing either generalized ill-effects or localized damage to the skin and surrounding tissues.

However carefully the scheme of treatment is devised, the tissues surrounding the growth are likely to suffer some temporary ill-effects and this is especially true of the skin. Therefore great care is required during and for some weeks after the treatment. The skin may be washed with soap and water, but it must be thoroughly dried without the use of vigorous rubbing. Graneodin ointment may be found soothing. If a male patient is receiving treatment to the face or neck, wet shaving is usually forbidden for a time, although dry shaving with an electric razor is allowed, and the friction of a closely fitting stiff collar should be avoided.

Mucous membranes react to radiation in much the same way as skin and some temporary damage to mucus-secreting cells will occur. If the mouth is included in the treatment area, there will be a diminution in the secretion of both saliva and mucus. The patient may be very disinclined to eat on account of the discomfort and pain caused by a dry mouth and must be helped and encouraged as much as possible. Frequent non-irritating fluids to drink and frequent mouth washes will help. If the mouth is painful, lozenges containing a local anaesthetic such as benzocaine may be ordered, or aspirin gargles may give relief.

General effects of radiation are not usually marked when divided dosage is used, spread over a period of weeks, but such effects were fairly common in the early days of X-ray treatment when a single large dose was used. However, some patients may complain of loss of appetite, nausea, diarrhoea, inability to sleep and general depression. It may be that some of these effects are due to the rapid disintegration of the mass of malignant cells.

Superficial application of X-rays is a method of treatment used for rodent ulcer and skin conditions such as keloid scars, and also occasionally in some conditions such as acne which have proved resistant to other forms of treatment. Treatment is usually planned in collaboration with the dermatologist and specific instructions will be given as to whether or not local applications are to be used at the same time.

Radium

Radium is a naturally-occurring element which spon-taneously emits various types of radiation of short wave-length. The penetrating radiations, known as gamma rays, are used therapeutically; the other radia-tions — alpha and beta rays — are screened off by the metal walls of the radium container. Radium is chiefly used in the form of its salt, radium sulphate, and in the form of the gas, radon, which is given off from it. The salt is placed in needles, gold 'grains' or larger con-tainers.

Methods of Application

Surface application   The needles or applicators are embedded in a suitable mould made of Columba paste, Perspex or Stent's dental composition, or may be attached to sorbo rubber or other suitable material which can be accurately applied to the desired area.

Interstitial irradiation   Needles or gold 'grains' are inserted into the tissues.

Cavity irradiation   Applicators are placed inside natu-ral cavities of the body, such as the vagina and cervical canal.

Rules and Precautions in Handling Radium

1. A standard symbol (Figure 11) has been adopted to denote the actual or potential presence of radiation and these signs are appropriately placed wherever there is a risk of contamination.

Figure 11. Radiation warning symbol

2. Radium needles or containers should never be touched by hand but must always be manipulated with long-handled forceps, the handles of which are covered with rubber. When radium is removed from the safe and carried to and from the theatre, a lead-lined box with a long carrying handle should be used.
3. The threading of needles and the preparation of applicators must be carried out on a special table provided with a lead screen.
4. Proximity to the radium must be for as short a time as possible.
5. The time at which the radium treatment is begun and the time at which it is due to be terminated must be carefully noted. The success of the treatment and the safety of the patient depend on careful calculation of the dosage to be employed. The time during which the radium is in contact with the tissues is one factor in these calculations.
6. Careful checking of the radium is essential. The theatre nurse or sister is responsible for checking the containers when brought to the theatre and

when removed from the sterilizer. The amount of radium, the number and the size of the needles used are entered on a record card; unused containers are checked and returned to the radium safe.

Radium is a valuable substance and careful checking at each stage is the best safeguard against accidental loss. Radium is also a dangerous substance; radium containers left about in the theatre or ward, or a radium needle that has slipped from its proper site and is lying in contact with healthy tissue, constitute a risk, in the one instance to the hospital personnel and in the other instance to the patient.

It is usual to issue rules for the guidance of those concerned with the care of radium and the nursing of patients undergoing radium treatment, and a disc showing the radiation symbol is attached to the bed. In the theatre a special card is filled in giving details of the number and type of needles and containers used, the time of insertion and of removal. This card is sent to the ward when the patient leaves the theatre and is completed when the radium is removed.

Radioactive Isotopes

Isotopes are variations of an element which have identical chemical properties but different atomic weights. Most elements have at least two isotopes. The radioactive isotopes of certain elements which are now being used in medical treatment are artificially produced by the bombardment of the nuclei of the atoms in an atomic pile. The radioactive isotopes used in medicine are, in fact, by-products of the atomic research stations. Examples of radioactive isotopes found to have a medical use include iodine, phosphorus, cobalt and gold.

Radioactive Iodine

This is used in the treatment of thyrotoxicosis and carcinoma of the thyroid gland. A measured dose is given by mouth and absorbed into the blood stream from the alimentary tract. From the blood it is deposited in the thyroid gland and there acts as a source of localized radiation. The iodine is given in sufficient dosage to obliterate excessive thyroid tissue or, in the case of carcinoma in patients over the age of 45, to destroy the malignant cells.

Radioactive Phosphorus

This has been found effective in the treatment of polycythaemia, a condition in which the blood contains an excessive number of red cells. The phosphorus may be given by mouth or by intravenous injection.

Radioactive Cobalt

This has a long 'life' compared with most other radioactive isotopes; it loses half its strength in rather more than five years. It is used in a beam unit and has an effect similar to that of high voltage X-ray therapy.

Radioactive Gold

This is used locally in the peritoneal or pleural cavities in cases of malignant disease where secondary deposits cause large peritoneal or pleural effusions necessitating frequent aspiration. The use of gold for this purpose has proved successful in reducing the effusion and thereby saving the patient considerable discomfort. Radioactive gold is also introduced into the peritoneal cavity after operation for a malignant condition if there is a possibility of an 'overspill' of malignant cells as, for example, from an ovarian cyst, or if minute deposits are known to be present in the peritoneum when the primary growth is removed.

Radioactive Tracers

Radioactive isotopes are useful assistants in solving physiological and medical problems. Very minute quantities can be traced in the body by means of a delicate instrument, the Geiger counter. If, for example, radioactive iodine is used, not for the treatment of disease of the thyroid gland but to assess the activity of the gland, a small dose is given by mouth and the Geiger counter is set up in position over the thyroid area and will record the arrival of the radioactive isotope in the tissues of the gland. If there is no active thyroid tissue no iodine will be taken up; if there is enlargement and/or increased activity of the gland the absorption of the iodine will be more rapid than normal. (See also p. 131.)

This ability to act as tracers in the body is proving to be one of the most important uses of radioactive isotopes.

Radiation Precautions

All persons working with radioactive substances or X-rays must observe the regulations laid down for their protection or their health will be affected. Prolonged exposure to even small doses of radiation will damage the bone marrow and eventually diminish the supply of blood cells. The ovaries and testes may be damaged by radiation resulting in sterility. In the early days of the use of X-rays, repeated exposure of the hands caused destruction of the skin, ulceration and later malignant changes. All staff working in radiography departments or with ionizing radiation carry monitoring film badges which record any exposure to radiation.

In the handling of radioactive isotopes, similar precautions are required as in dealing with other forms of radiation, but in addition there is the danger of contamination with radioactive particles. If the worker's hands become contaminated there is danger of swallowing these particles. Radioactive dust may also be inhaled during the course of the work. Therefore, in addition to working behind protective screens, protective clothing, including rubber gloves, is worn. Handling radioactive material is carried out by means of long-handled tools and instruments. It is of course essential that no eating, drinking or smoking should be allowed during such work.

When patients are receiving doses of radioactive iodine, some of the material will be excreted in the urine, most of it within the first 48 hours. Typical regulations are as follows:

1. Areas of treated skin may be washed with soap and water but must be thoroughly dried.
2. The patient is given frequent non-irritating fluids to drink and mouth washes of glycerin and thymol.
3. Asprin or paracetamol will relieve soreness of mouth and throat, and lignocaine spray may be used to rinse the mouth.
4. Graneodin ointment may be used for external application.
5. Palpation and washing of the neck should be avoided.
6. Patients are required to use one designated toilet which should be flushed twice after use and monitored periodically.
7. When a bedpan or urinal is used, it should be

emptied immediately and then washed and rinsed with sodium iodide, avoiding splashing. Rubber gloves must be worn.

Vomit   Bowls used in the first 24 hours should be emptied and washed, then placed in plastic bags and stored until monitoring is possible.

Faeces   No precautions are required.

Hands   To avoid contamination of the hands, rubber gloves are worn when attending to an incontinent patient receiving therapeutic radiation. Gloves should be washed on the hands before they are removed. The hands must be washed after removing the gloves, and again before eating or smoking.

In the case of smaller, tracer doses of radioactive material these stringent precautions are not considered necessary. Contaminated equipment, clothing and bed linen should be handled with rubber gloves, placed in plastic bags and stored outside the ward until taken away by the staff of the physics department.

20
Food Requirements

The normal daily diet should contain proteins, carbohydrates and fats, for energy, growth and repair, in the following proportions:

Protein — 10–15% of the whole. (This should be, on average, 1 g per kg of body weight.)
Carbohydrate — 50–60% of the whole.
Fat — 30–35% of the whole.

In addition, the body needs water, vitamins and salts. These are usually present in sufficient quantities for health in the average mixed diet. Thirst is normally an adequate guide to fluid intake, but at least 2 litres per day are required in addition to the water obtained from foods and from oxidation of food in the body.

Energy Requirements

Energy requirements of the body are measured in units of energy known as kilojoules (kJ). One kilojoule is the amount of energy required to raise the temperature of 1 kg of water, i.e. 1 litre, by 1°C. One gram of protein yields 16.7 kJ, as does 1 g of carbohydrate, while 1 g of fat gives 37.6 kJ. The energy value of various foods can therefore be calculated with reasonable accuracy.

Standardized tables are available in which the energy requirement can be quickly found for any person whose weight, height and age are known. The average daily energy requirements for adults and children are shown in Table VII in both kilojoules and kilocalories (Calories).

The *basal metabolic requirement* is the minimum

Table VII. Average daily energy requirements

	Energy requirements				
	Male		Female		
	kJ	kcal	kJ	kcal	
Adult (70 kg man, 56 kg woman)					
Sedentary (150 kJ/kg)	10 500	2 510	8 400	2 010	
Active (180 kJ/kg)	12 600	3 015	10 080	2 410	
Very active (267 kJ/kg)	18 690	4 470	14 950	3 575	
Child					
Aged 1 year	4 285	1 025	4 285	1 025	
3 years	6 000	1 435	6 000	1 435	
5 years	7 525	1 800	7 525	1 800	
10 years	10 115	2 420	9 400	2 250	
14 years	12 540	3 000	9 825	2 350	
15 years	13 795	3 300	10 660	2 550	

N.B. To convert kilojoules to kilocalories (Calories) divide by 4·18, i.e. 1 kcal = 4·18 kJ.

amount of energy needed to sustain bodily functions, such as respiration and cardiac output, during complete physical rest or sleep. More than half the energy obtained from the daily food intake is required for basal metabolic activity, i.e. about 7524 kJ for an average healthy adult male and 6270 kJ for the healthy adult female.

Pregnancy and Lactation

During the latter half of pregnancy and during lactation the mother's diet needs to be adequate but not excessive; a daily intake of 10 500–12 500 kJ (2500–3000 calories) may be regarded as meeting average requirements. The protein proportion should be increased to 1.5 g per kg of body weight.

Other additional daily requirements are:
  Iron (15–20 mg).
  Vitamin A (6000 International Units).
  Vitamin D (600 International Units).   .

Diet in Illness

The factors which alter the body's requirements during illness should influence the choice of diet for the patient. Because he is lying inactive in bed his calorie requirements will not necessarily be small. For example, trauma to the body tissues as a result of burns, accidents, surgery or infection will result in excessive loss of protein and the nurse must see that protein in excess of normal requirements is supplied. The permeability of blood capillaries may be affected if vitamin C is short in the diet so this must be included in sufficient quantities as a good blood supply is a prerequisite of tissue healing. At the time of admission, or subsequently, a patient's emotional state may inhibit the secretion of gastric juice, so affecting his digestion. He should be reassured and helped to feel relaxed and self-confident. Presentation, size of helping and digestibility of the food offered may restore his appetite.

A knowledge of energy requirements alone is insufficient; the diet should be balanced to include the essential nutrients in the right proportion to each other and to the metabolic needs of the patient. Carbohydrates may supply sufficient energy but will not meet the nutritional needs of a growing child or a patient who requires extra protein or vitamin C. Tables are issued by the Department of Health showing the amounts of the different nutrients needed in health and in illness. Tables are also available stating either the proportion of the diet or the minimum intake of carbohydrate, protein and fats in relation to the needs of the patient.

Dietetics is the science of regulating diet. In hospital it can be applied successfully in relation to particular diseases, e.g. the carbohydrate intake is regulated in the treatment of diabetes mellitus. Most hospitals have trained dieticians and a special kitchen where the many different diets are prepared. Some diets may prove unpopular with the patient, e.g. a reducing diet. The nurse can do much to help the patient accept his diet by explaining its function in meeting his particular needs and by seeing that it is served promptly and attractively. The nurse must be able to offer an alternative of equivalent dietary value if a patient cannot accept a specific item of food on religious grounds.

A knowledge of nutrition equips the nurse, as a health teacher, to help her patients with various problems associated not only with the diet in disease but also good diet as a means of preventing illness.

Nasogastric Feeding

When the diet has to be supplied in fluid form, for example to an unconscious patient, proprietary foods are available containing the essential constituents in concentrated form. These are administered via a nasogastric tube. Initially it must be established that the stomach can empty properly. Ideally a Ryle's tube should be passed and calculated amounts of water given via the tube; throughout the first 24-hour period the stomach should be aspirated every four hours, a diminished return showing that absorption is taking place. Following this, the Ryle's tube is removed, and a 1 mm (fine) bore nasogastric tube is passed into the stomach using a fine guide wire. Once this tube is in position the guide wire is removed and the nasogastric tube is attached to a prepared intragastric drip feed. The greater the volume prepared, the less nursing time is spent in changing the drip feed; volumes of 500 ml, 1 litre or 3 litres are commonly used. The use of the fine bore tube reduces many of the discomforts which result from the larger, less flexible Ryle's tube, and diarrhoea is less frequent using continuous intragastric drip feeding than with intermittent feeding methods. When patients are receiving tube feeds over a long period of time, daily observations of urine volume, stool frequency and, if possible, weight should be carried out. The fluid dietary regimen can also be monitored by regular checks on the blood glucose, urinary electrolytes and urea, packed cell volume, haemoglobin, and blood urea.

The following proprietary foods are commonly used to prepare intragastric feeds: Clinifeed, Caloreen, Casilan and Complan. If the nasogastric route cannot be used, intravenous parenteral therapy may be necessary (see p. 59).

Table VIII. Vitamin chart

Vitamin	Functions and Deficiency Effects	Good Natural Sources	Optimum Daily Requirements
A Fat soluble Slowly destroyed by exposure to air or light Rapidly destroyed by rancidity or fat	Necessary for health and growth, by maintaining healthy mucous membranes and skin and for the normal functioning of the visual purple in the eye *Deficiency Effects* *Mild:* Lowered resistance to infection, night blindness *Severe:* Xerophthalmia, infection of the mucous membranes	Fish, liver oils, most meats, butter, cheese, oily fish, margarine, green vegetables, carrots, tomatoes, apricots	*Infants to Adolescents* 1000–5000 IU *Adults* 3000 IU *Pregnant and lactating women* 6000–8000 IU
B-complex All water-soluble			
B1 *Aneurin* Anti-neuritic	Concerned with cell respiration and carbohydrate metabolism *Deficiency Effects* *Mild:* Loss of appetite, digestive disturbances, debility, retarded growth, nervous disorders, insomnia *Severe:* Beri beri, polyneuritis	Almost all foods except white flour and sugar	About 1·5–2 mg

B2
Riboflavine
Less stable when exposed to light

Like B1, B2 forms a link in the chain of processes through which the body obtains energy from carbohydrates and is necessary for healthy skin

Deficiency Effects
Mild: Digestive disturbances, burning and soreness of the eyes, lips and tongue, weakness, retarded growth
Severe: Diarrhoea, dermatitis, loss of hair, sores at the angle of the mouth, corneal opacities

Milk, eggs, cheese, liver, kidney, yeast, wholemeal bread

Children: 1·5 mg
Adults: 1·5–2 mg

B6
Pyridoxine
Unstable in light

Concerned with protein metabolism and healthy skin

Unpolished rice or rice bran, whole cereals, yeast, milk, liver, wheat germ, small amounts in most foods

10–20 mg

B12
Cyanocobalamin

Ensures blood cell development in the bone marrow in combination with folic acid.
Deficiency may lead to pernicious anaemia and nerve cell degeneration

Animal products only, e.g. liver, cheese, eggs, beef, white fish. Deficiency unlikely if eating a mixed diet. Vegans require to supplement their diet.

Table VIII. Vitamin chart *(continued)*

Vitamin	Functions and Deficiency Effects	Good Natural Sources	Optimum Daily Requirements
Nicotinic Acid Anti-pellagra	Functions similar to that of ribo-flavine (B2). May be used thera-peutically to cause vasodilation *Deficiency Effects* *Mild*: Loss of weight, sore tongue, mouth infections, rough red skin especially parts exposed to light *Severe*: Pellagra (symptoms of diarrhoea, dermatitis, dementia)	Meat, whole cereals, yeast, bacon	10–20 mg
Pantothenic Acid *Biotin*	Health of skin	} as for B12	
Folic acid	Similar to vitamin B12 Used in the treatment of macrocytic anaemia		

C *Ascorbic acid* Water-soluble Unstable to heat but rapid cooking less destructive than long, slow cooking. No destruction in modern canning of fruit and vegetables	Necessary for production of normal endothelial and epithelial cells and for growth *Deficiency Effects* *Mild:* Slow healing of wounds and fractures, anaemia, infection of mouth and gums *Severe:* Scurvy (tender swollen extremities, subcutaneous and submucous haemorrhages)	Fresh fruit and vegetables, black-currant juice either fresh or sold in bottles bearing on the label the amount of vitamin C present	30–50 mg
D *Calciferol* Anti-rachitic Fat-soluble	Regulates metabolism of calcium and phosphorus, necessary for growth of bones and teeth *Deficiency Effects* *Mild:* Poor muscle tone, retarded skeletal growth *Severe:* Rickets, Osteomalacia	Fish-liver oils, eggs, butter, margarine Vitamin D can also be produced in the body by exposure to sunlight or ultra-violet light	*Infants, pregnant and lactating women:* 600–800 IU *Children:* 400 IU *Adults:* 200 IU

Table VIII. Vitamin chart *(continued)*

Vitamin	Functions and Deficiency Effects	Good Natural Sources	Optimum Daily Requirements
E Fat-soluble	The functions of this particular vitamin are as yet uncertain, although it may be used to produce peripheral vasodilation	Wheat germ oil, oats, milk, green leaves and lettuce	
K Anti-haemorrhagic Fat-soluble	Essential for maintaining the normal blood-clotting function Bile is necessary for the absorption of vitamin K, therefore deficiency is often associated with obstructive jaundice and diseases of the liver *Deficiency Effects* Prolonged bleeding and clotting times	Deficiency unlikely if eating a well-balanced diet	

Vitamins

Vitamins are regarded as essential for growth and health, although it is difficult to define accurately the part played by some of them in normal development and in the maintenance of health. Most modern diets contain adequate vitamins and only the young, the aged and the pregnant woman are likely to need vitamin supplements. Only enough vitamins should be given to improve the patient's condition to a point where a normal diet will supply all the remaining necessary nutrients.

Vitamins can be given in the form of tablets or capsules for oral administration or by injection. Vitamin K may be given prophylactically to people undergoing surgery if they have a tendency to bleed excessively, or to patients receiving anticoagulant drugs if they should start to bleed.

A list of the most important vitamins, their properties, the effect of deficiency, natural sources in food and the optimum daily intake of each, is given in Table VIII (pp. 146–150).

Minerals

The main requirements are calcium, copper, iodine, iron, phosphorus, potassium and sodium. The biological properties and natural sources of these elements are given in Table IX.

Table IX.   Mineral inorganic elements

Name	Biological properties	Good natural sources
Calcium	Necessary for all body processes, particularly bone and teeth formation during years of growth. An essential constituent of blood *Daily needs:* in pregnancy 1.5 g; in childhood/adolescence 1–1.4 g; in adults 1g	Milk, milk products, especially cheese, dried milk; egg yolk, green leafy vegetables, especially outer leaves, oats, rice, wheat, legumes, nuts, coconut, citrus fruits, dried figs, lettuce, carrots, sardines
Copper	Speeds up formation of haemoglobin of red blood cells Very minute amount needed	Sufficient amounts present in any well-balanced diet
Iodine	Minute amounts needed by thyroid gland in making thyroxine	Water, fish, vegetables. Iodized table salt can supplement natural sources
Iron	Essential constituent of haemoglobin in red blood cells *Average daily need:* 10–15 mg	Meat, liver, kidneys, egg yolk, fish, especially salt-water fish, oat meal, black treacle, maize, rice, wheat, legumes, nuts, coconut, dried figs, carrots, green and yellow vegetables and fruits. In apples, peaches and apricots the iron lies just under the skin.

Table IX. Mineral inorganic elements *(continued)*

Name	Biological properties	Good natural sources
Phosphorus	Needed for normal function of cells; for bones and teeth, calcium phosphate being the chief inorganic constituent of bone Amount contained in a mixed diet is ample	Meat, fish, liver, brains, pancreas, etc., milk, dried milk, cheese, egg yolk, barley, kaffir-corn, maize, millet, oats, rice, wheat, legumes, nuts, coconut, plums, dried figs, lettuce, carrots, cocoa
Potassium	Essential constituent of the body cells	Present in many substances in a normal diet
Sodium	Constituent of body cells and fluids Most abundant in extracellular fluid 5 g daily should be ample More salt is needed in hot climates where loss of water and salt through sweating is increased	Sodium (sodium chloride) is the only salt eaten as such Found in all animal cells, e.g. meat, and present in most foods as part of their chemical make-up

21
SI Units

The SI system was formally introduced in December 1975 and has replaced the previous Imperial system of weights and measures used in the United Kingdom. Nursing has joined many other professions in expressing scientific measurements in the same language. Table X illustrates the SI system of prefixes to indicate different-sized units. Several features are to be noted. The abbreviated symbols must always be written as shown; notice that mega (M) is expressed using the capital letter whereas all other symbols use small letters. The old abbreviation mcg (microgram) can be confused with mg (milligram) and

Table X. SI prefixes

Prefix	Symbol	Multiple	Example	Index
mega	M	1000 000	1 megawatt (MW) = 1000 000 watts (W)	10^6
kilo	k	1000	1 kilogram (kg) = 1000 grams (g)	10^3
centi	c	1/100	1 centimetre (cm) = 1/100 metre (m)	10^{-2}
milli	m	1/1000	1 milligram (mg) = 1/1000 gram (g)	10^{-3}
micro	μ	1/1000 000	1 microgram (μg) = 1/1000 000 gram (g)	10^{-6}
nano	n	1/1000 000 000	1 nanogram (ng) = 1/1000 000 000 gram (g)	10^{-9}
pico	p	1/1000 000 000 000	1 picogram (pg) = 1/1000 000 000 000 gram (g)	10^{-12}

medical staff should write 'micrograms' out in full on prescriptions. The standard SI symbol for microgram is μg.

The digits of large numbers are grouped together in threes and commas should never be used since they may be mistaken for decimal points. Should results involving the use of large numbers be given over the telephone, each digit should be spoken separately, the word zero used instead of nought, and the complete result read back for a double check.

Pathology departments reduce large numbers by the use of indices as shown in the last column of Table X. Compare the 'multiple' column with 'index' column. The multiple 1000 can be expressed as 10^3 because $1000 = 10 \times 10 \times 10$. This reduces the effort and possible error in writing and reading large numbers. A further example is =

$10^6 = 10 \times 10 \times 10 \times 10 \times 10 \times 10$, which gives us 1 and six zeros, i.e. 1 000 000 or 1 million.

Where the multiple is a fraction, 1/1000 for example, the index is negative. $1/1000 = 1 \div (10 \times 10 \times 10)$, which is written as 10^{-3}. As a decimal this is 0.001, i.e. 10^{-3} has the 1 in the third place after the decimal point. Similarly $10^{-6} = 0.000 001$.

The simple rules to follow when interpreting such figures are therefore:
1. 10 with a positive index; the index indicates the number of zeros following the 1.
2. 10 with a negative index; the index indicates the place of the figure 1 after the decimal point.

When using a decimal point, make it clear and always fill in the blank space preceding a decimal point with a zero, e.g. .5 should be written 0.5.

Units of Volume

16–17 drops = 1 millilitre (ml)
1000 ml   = 1 litre (l)

Units of Weight

1 kilogram (kg) = 1000 grams (g)
1 g   = 1000 milligrams (mg)
1 mg   = 1000 micrograms (μg)

Units of Length

1 kilometre (km) = 1000 metres (m)
1 m   = 100 centimetres (cm)
1 cm   = 10 millimetres (mm)

Approximate Domestic Measurements

Medicines dispensed by chemists are clearly labelled
with instructions for the patient's guidance and all oral
mixtures are dispensed with a 5 ml spoon so that
mistakes by the patient are kept to a minimum.
However, at home approximate measurements using
domestic crockery are sometimes a safe and satisfactory alternative.

    Average-sized tumbler = approx. 200 ml
    Average-sized teacup   = approx. 150 ml
    Dessertspoon   = approx. 7–10 ml

Calculating a Dosage

Dosages expressed in the SI system are usually
straightforward, but occasionally a more difficult dosage is prescribed.

Example: The ampoule of the drug contains 250 mg in 2 ml and the dose prescribed is 100 mg.

250 mg are contained in 2 ml,

therefore 1 mg is contained in $\dfrac{2}{250}$ ml,

100 mg are contained in $100 \times \dfrac{2}{250}$ ml,

$$= \dfrac{200}{250} \text{ ml} = \dfrac{4}{5} \text{ ml}.$$

Percentage Solutions

'Percentage' is used to denote the strength of a solution. The percentage may be weight in volume (W/V) or volume in volume (V/V) depending on the solution. W/V solution means that the solute is a solid which must be measured in weight, whereas the solvent is a liquid and must be measured in volume units. V/V solution means that both the solute and the solvent are liquids and both are therefore measured in volume units.

A volume % is also used to express the amount of gas dissolved in a liquid. For example, when 10 ml of gas is dissolved in 100 ml of fluid the concentration can be expressed as 10% (V/V).

A 1% solution prepared according to the metric system is equivalent to 1 g in 100 ml of solution.

Dilution of Lotions

Where instructions are not supplied regarding the necessary dilution factor, the following formula can be used to find how much stock solution is required:

$$\text{Vol. of stock soln} = \frac{\text{Strength required}}{\text{Strength of stock solution}}$$

$$\times \text{ Vol. required}$$

This formula may be abbreviated to:

$$\frac{\text{I Want}}{\text{I Have}} \times \text{Vol. required} = \text{Amount stock soln required}$$

Example: To prepare 600 ml of 1-in-30 solution from a stock solution of 1-in-10.

$$\text{Vol. of stock needed} = \frac{1/30}{1/10} \times 600$$

(To divide by the fraction 1/10 turn it upside down and multiply by 10/1.)

$$= 1/30 \times 10/1 \times 600$$
$$= 200 \text{ ml of stock solution.}$$

As 600 ml of 1-in-30 solution is required, 400 ml of water must be added to the 200 ml of stock solution to produce 600 ml of solution at a dilution of 1-in-30.

This method can also be used when the ratios are expressed as percentages. To express a ratio as a percent, multiply by 100.

Example: 1-in-20 ratio $= 1/20 \times 100 = \dfrac{100}{20} = 5\%$

To express a percentage as a ratio, divide by 100.

Example: $20\% = 20/100 = 1/5 = 1\text{-in-}5$

If the problem includes both a ratio and a percentage, convert one to the other.

Example: To prepare 400 ml of 0·02% solution from a 1-in-200 stock solution.

1-in-200 as a % is $1/200 \times 100 = \frac{1}{2} = 0·5\%$

Vol. of stock needed

$$= \frac{\%\ \text{strength required}}{\%\ \text{strength of stock}} \times \text{vol. required}$$

$$= \frac{0·02}{0·5} \times 400 \quad = 16\ \text{ml}$$

The amount of water required is therefore
400 − 16 = 384 ml
i.e. 16 ml of stock solution + 384 ml of water gives 400 ml of 0.02 solution.

Thermometric Scale

The fundamental unit for measuring temperature is the degree Kelvin, but in clinical work body temperature is measured in degrees Celsius (°C) which are identical to degrees Centigrade. The term 'Centigrade' should no longer be used since it refers to the French unit for measuring angles.

0°C	= the temperature of melting ice at sea level.
100°C	= the temperature of steam given off when water is boiled under atmospheric pressure at sea level.
36–37°C	= the average human physiological body temperature.

At 35°C and below a patient is regarded as hypothermic.

At 37.2°C and above a patient is regarded as being pyrexial.

Thermometers

Clinical   For normal use; has a scale from 35 to 45°C.

Rectal   A similar range of scale but distinguished by an elongated (usually blue) mercurial bulb.

Low-reading   This has a scale between 25 and 40°C and is used in suspected cases of hypothermia, e.g. when elderly people are admitted in winter or in an obviously neglected state, and in some cases of hypothyroidism.

Electronic thermometers   These are available for highly specialized work such as induced hypothermia. They are passed into the nasopharynx, oesophagus, trachea, skin or muscle and attached by leads to an electric recording machine for continuous monitoring.

Disposable thermometers   These are available for use in isolation nursing and have the same scale as the clinical thermometer.

Temperatures for Irrigations

Lotions for swabbing wounds and irrigating body cavities should be used at 38°C unless there are instructions to the contrary.

Syringing the external auditory meatus with lotion that is hotter or colder than the body temperature will stimulate the semicircular canals of the internal ear and may cause giddiness and nausea.

The temperature of bathing water for infants should be 38°C.

'Tepid sponging' is a prescribed therapy. The temperature of the water is usually about 30°C at the commencement and this is gradually reduced to roughly 24°C. If very cold sponging is ordered, the water should be kept as near 0°C as possible by the addition of ice.

Other Measurements in the SI System

The term 'Hertz' replaces 'cycles per second'. For example, the frequency of vibration of a tuning fork which vibrates at 300 cycles per second will now be expressed as 300 Hertz (Hz).

Energy and heat may be measured in joules rather than calories. The joule is smaller than the calorie; 1 calorie = 4.2 joules. However, the kilocalorie or Calorie used in dietetics equals 4200 joules (4.2 kJ).

The term 'mole' denotes the amount of a substance in terms of the number of molecular particles present. The mole replaces other ways of describing the weight of a substance in solution (e.g. in body fluids) of interest in biochemistry and pharmacy. The term 'mole' allows chemical quantities to be correctly expressed in terms of their fundamental reacting particles. Because the mole is too large a unit for clinical use, most values will be expressed as millimoles (mmol), a millimole being 1/1000 of a mole. Smaller units are also available (see Table X on p. 154).

1 mole = 1000 millimoles (mmol); 1 mmol = 10^{-3} mol

1 mmol = 1000 micromoles (μmol); 1 μmol = 10^{-6} mol

$1\mu\text{mol} = 1000$ nanomoles (nmol); 1 nmol $= 10^{-9}$ mol

1 nmol $= 1000$ picomoles (pmol); 1 pmol $= 10^{-12}$ mol

For example:

Blood glucose is expressed in mmol/litre.

Serum bilirubin is expressed in μmol/litre.

Thyroxine is expressed in nmol/litre.

Thryoid-stimulating hormone is expressed in pmol/litre.

22
The Examination of Urine

Collection of a Specimen

Usually a specimen of urine passed on waking in the early morning is required for routine ward testing. However, if a patient is admitted to hospital as an urgent case, a specimen of urine is collected as soon as possible. The first early morning specimen of urine passed by a diabetic patient should be discarded, as urine which has accumulated in the bladder during the night does not give an accurate result.

Specimens should be collected into clean dry containers, which have not been contaminated with detergents or disinfectants which may affect some of the chemical tests. Whether in the ward or the laboratory, testing should be carried out with freshly passed urine; if the specimen is allowed to stand, decomposition begins and important constituents may be altered or destroyed.

Specimens for Bacteriological Examination

These specimens are collected into sterile containers and aseptic precautions are observed. In the case of a woman patient a catheter specimen may be required. Catherization, however careful the aseptic technique may be, carries some risk of infection and a 'clean' specimen of urine may be considered suitable for both male and female patients.

To collect a 'clean' specimen of urine The external genitalia are thoroughly washed with soap and water. The area around the urethral orifice is swabbed with a suitable mildly antiseptic lotion, and swabbed dry. The patient is then asked to pass the first part of the urinary stream into the toilet or bedpan. A sample of the middle of the urinary stream is then collected into the container and the patient concludes micturition into the toilet. The collection of 'clean' specimens of urine from infants and toddlers is best accomplished by attaching an adhesive Uri-bag around the genitalia.

To Collect a 24-hour Specimen of Urine

At a specific, noted time, e.g. 8 a.m., the patient is asked to empty his bladder and the urine is discarded. All urine passed during the ensuing 24 hours is collected into a large container provided by the laboratory. At 8 a.m. the following day the patient is asked to empty the bladder and this urine is added to the container, completing the specimen. If possible, patients should be made responsible for their own collections, provided the bed carries a warning notice of the specimen collection. Careful labelling of the container is the nurse's responsibility.

Routine Ward Observations

Volume   An adult in health excretes about 1–1.5 litres of urine per 24 hours, but this can vary considerably, being influenced by variations in the fluid intake and the loss of fluid by other routes such as sweating. In some diseases the urinary output increases (polyuria); for example in chronic renal failure when the kidney is unable to concentrate the urine, diabetes mellitus where the amount of urine increases in order to dilute and excrete glucose (which is not normally present in urine), and diabetes insipidus, a condition in which the pituitary glands fail to produce the water retaining (antidiuretic) hormone. Decrease in the urinary output (oliguria) occurs in nephritis, acute renal failure, any condition which reduces the blood supply to the kidneys, circulatory failure from any cause, and cardiac failure. Certain toxic chemicals, such as sulphonamides, arsenical compounds and mercury, also produce oliguria by damaging the kidney. *Accurate* measurement of the volume of urine passed is essential in many pathological conditions.

Colour Urine is usually described as pale amber, but the colour varies according to the concentration of the particular specimen observed. Very dilute urine is almost colourless, while concentrated urine is dark yellow.

The colour is altered by the presence of some abnormal constituents. A significant amount of blood will colour the urine red or a smoky-brown; bile gives it a greenish-brown colour. Dyes excreted in the urine can also alter the colour. For example, the urine appears blue after the administration of indigo-carmine or Diagnex Blue, a cation-exchange resin; blackcurrant juice or beetroot taken in sufficient quantities will colour the urine red.

Deposits When urine is collected in a specimen glass and allowed to stand, a deposit can usually be seen which is due to the precipitation of normal urinary constituents — urates and phosphates.

Mucus, pus, red blood cells and epithelial casts from the renal tubules are some of the abnormal substances which may form a deposit. In such cases the deposit is usually required for microscopic examination.

Specific gravity   The specific gravity of a substance is the weight of 1 litre of that substance compared with the weight of 1 litre of distilled water, which is 1000 g. The specific gravity of normal urine varies from 1.003 to 1.030, varying with fluid intake and fluid loss which affect the concentration of the urine. A high specific gravity and large volume of urine is found in diabetes mellitus, due to the presence of sugar. A persistently low specific gravity is one of the signs of renal failure.

Routine ward tests for specific gravity are regarded as being merely indicative. A more accurate test completed in the laboratory would involve freezing a specific volume of urine; the amount by which the freezing point is below that of water is determined by the amount of solute in the urine.

Reactions   Normal urine is usually slightly acid, although urine passed immediately after a meal may be alkaline. If a specimen of urine is left to stand it will become alkaline, owing to the conversion of urea into ammonia. Litmus paper is commonly used to test the reaction of a specimen of urine. Acid urine turns blue litmus paper red. Alkaline urine turns red litmus paper blue. Neutral urine does not alter the colour of either red or blue litmus.

Abnormal Constituents

Proteins   Plasma proteins do not normally pass from the blood in to the urine, but may do so when the renal tubules are damaged, for example in acute nephritis, the nephrotic syndrome and damage due to toxins. Proteinuria (albuminuria) may also be present in acute febrile conditions and congestive heart failure. Occasionally it occurs in healthy young adults; protein appears in the urine at the end of the day, but after a night's rest it disappears. This condition, which is known as 'postural proteinuria', is not usually associated with any disease process and clears up spontaneously.

Glucose   The presence of glucose in the urine is usually an indication of diabetes mellitus. However, it is occasionally due to other hormone disturbances or to a non-pathological condition in which the renal threshold for glucose is lower than normal, when the kidneys may excrete some glucose following the intake of a considerable quantity of carbohydrate.

Acetone and diacetic acid   These ketone bodies are formed and excreted as a result of the incomplete metabolism of fats associated with some abnormality of carbohydrate metabolism. In diabetes mellitus the presence of acetone and diacetic acid in the urine is a warning of the possibility of diabetic coma.

Blood   Blood may be found in the urine of patients suffering from disease or injury of the urinary tract, e.g. acute nephritis, renal or bladder stones, tumours, bilharzial infestation, tuberculosis of the kidney, or crush injuries involving the kidney or bladder.

Bile   Bile is present in the urine in cases of obstructive jaundice, e.g. a gall stone in the common bile duct, and in inflammatory diseases of the liver, e.g. infective hepatitis.

Pus   Pus may be found in the urine in any infection of the urinary tract, in cystitis, pyelitis, in association with renal calculi and also in tuberculous infection.

Testing Urine

It is now common practice for proprietary reagent strips and tablets to be used for the testing of urine. Some of these demonstrate the presence of abnormal constituents whilst others indicate the quantity. Strips impregnated with several reagents permit several tests to be performed simultaneously.

Clear instructions and colour charts are issued for these different tests. If they are not followed meticulously, with regard to the number of drops of urine and/or water to be used and the exact timing for observations, inaccuracies may result. A standardized test tube and dropper must also be used in conjunction with these products and filter paper must not be substituted for the test maps as the texture is incorrect. When a colour comparison is to be made, it is important that the colour chart is held close enough to the test. It is not necessary during these particular tests to filter the urine or to acidify it, but one must still avoid testing stale alkaline urine.

It is customary in out-patient clinics and on first admitting a patient to test first for the presence of abnormalities. Where abnormalities are detected quantitive tests are performed before reporting the result to the doctor.

Routine Screening Tests

Using Multiple Strips:

N-Multistix	Test for pH, protein, glucose, ketones, bilirubin, blood, nitrite and urobilinogen
Multistix	Test for pH, protein, glucose, ketones, bilirubin, blood and urobilinogen

N-Labstix	Test for pH, protein, glucose, ketones, blood and nitrite

Using Single Strips:

Litmus paper or pH indicator	Test for pH
Albustix	Test for protein
Diastix, Clinistix	Test for glucose (Diastix is specific for glucose and more sensitive than Clinitest)
Ketostix, Acetest	Test for ketones
Ictotest	Test for bilirubin
Hemastix	Test for blood

Diabetic Tests

Clinitest	Copper reduction test, sensitive to all reducing sugars such as lactose, fructose, and demonstrating a quantity of 0–2% (or 5% if two-drop method used)
Keto-Diastix	Test for glucose and ketones
Diastix	Test for glucose
Ketostix	Test for ketones

Hepato/biliary Tests

Urobilistix	Test for urobilinogen
Ictotest	Test for bilirubin

Phenylketone Tests

Phenistix   The instructions issued with these strips should be observed carefully as positive results may be masked when certain drugs have been administered. Although this is unlikely in babies, the tests may be used for adults in mental hospitals who may be receiving drug treatment.

23
Laboratory Investigations

Laboratory investigations play a large part in modern medicine. They vary greatly in their complexity and significance, but most of them depend for their success not only upon the laboratory work but also upon the care and accuracy with which the specimens are collected and transmitted to the laboratory. It is therefore useful for the nurse to have some knowledge of the nature and purpose of these tests.

Collection of Samples

All specimens sent to the laboratory should be as fresh as possible, for in many cases even a few hours delay will render the specimen unsuitable for examination, due to bacterial decomposition or other causes.

Specimens should, if possible, be collected first thing in the morning before breakfast, because the taking of a meal may affect the level of some substances in the blood or urine. Taking and delivering specimens to the laboratory in the morning is also very helpful to the laboratory staff to enable them to organize their work load. All specimens should be clearly labelled to prevent loss.

Bacteriological Examination

In many conditions specimens are required for bacteriological examination in order to identify the microorganism responsible. Such specimens include throat, nose and wound swabs, sputum, stools, pleural and cerebrospinal fluids. These specimens must be collected under strict aseptic conditions and in sterile containers. An exception to this is the collection of faeces; the entire stool may be sent to the laboratory in the bed-pan (labelled) in which it is passed, or a small quantity of the material (particularly mucus, pus and blood if present) may be sent to the laboratory in a screw-capped container.

When taking swabs for bacteriological examination, care must be taken to ensure that no antiseptic is applied to the surface for several hours prior to swabbing. If the patient is being treated with a chemotherapeutic agent, this should be stated on the pathology request form. All specimens will be examined by direct smear and culture; information can also be obtained with regard to the sensitivity of organisms to various antibiotics.

Specimens of Blood

When sending blood for examination the greatest care must be taken to avoid haemolysis of the specimen, for haemolysis almost invariably renders it unusable. For some tests blood serum is required, whilst for others whole unclotted blood must be sent. To prevent clotting, potassium oxalate or sodium citrate is added to the specimen containers. The hospital laboratory usually recommends the use of standard specimen containers, and in some areas phlebotomists are employed to take blood and be responsible for its delivery to the laboratory.

Blood test	Amount and type of blood required
Absolute indices	2–5 ml sequestrene
Acid phosphatase	5 ml clotted
Alcohol	2.5 ml clotted or sequestrene
Alkali reserve	*5 ml

Alkaline phosphatase	5 ml clotted
Amylase	5 ml clotted
Antibody (antenatal test)	8–10 ml clotted
Antistreptolysin titre (ASOT)	10 ml clotted
Barbiturates	10 ml heparinized
Berger Kahn (Kahn)	8–10 ml clotted
Bilirubin	5–10 ml clotted (see p. 186)
Blood count	2–3 ml sequestrene
Bromide	10 ml clotted
Bromsulphthalein	10 ml clotted (see p. 187)
Brucella agglutination	5–10 ml clotted
C reactive protein	3–5 ml clotted
Calcium	5 ml clotted
Chloride	5 ml clotted
Cholesterol	5 ml oxalated
Cold agglutins	5 ml clotted (despatch within 15 minutes of collection)
Coombs	5 ml clotted
Electrolytes	5 ml heparinized
Erythrocyte sedimentation rate	2–3 ml sequestrene
Fibrinogen	2–3 ml sequestrene
Folic acid	15–20 ml clotted
Gonococcal complement fixation	*5–10 ml
Grouping and cross-matching	2–5 ml sequestrene +10 ml clotted
Lactic dehydrogenase (LDH)	5 ml clotted
Lipase	10 ml clotted
Packed cell volume	2–5 ml sequestrene
Paul Bunnell	5 ml clotted
Potassium	*5 ml
Protein	5 ml clotted
Protein-bound iodine	*10 ml

(see p. 186)
(see p. 187)

Prothrombin	*2–5 ml
Pyruvic acid	*10 ml
RA latex agglutinations	3–5 ml clotted
Salicylate	5 ml clotted
AST (SGOT) and	
ALT (SGPT)	5 ml clotted
Sodium	*5 ml
Thyocyanate	7 ml clotted
Thymol turbidity	2 ml clotted
Thyroid antibody	5 ml clotted
Toxoplasma dye	10 ml clotted
Treponema immobili-	
zation (TPI)	*10 ml
Urea	2–5 ml sequestrene
Uric acid	5 ml clotted
van den Bergh	5 ml clotted
Viruses and Rickettsiae	10 ml clotted + a second specimen taken 10–14 days later
Vitamin B12	15–20 ml clotted
Wassermann reaction	*10 ml

*denotes that the laboratory will provide a special container for this specimen.

If there is any doubt as to the amount or type of blood required for any specimen, the laboratory should be contacted for advice. In the larger laboratories using computerized systems the above list may prove inadequate.

A number of tests are carried out by the laboratory staff on the wards, and on these occasions they will bring their own equipment. Such tests include:

Astrup (*the buffering power of the blood*), which may also include the alkali reserve.
Bilirubin from Rhesus babies.

Blood culture.
Sternal marrow puncture.
Synacthen stimulation test.

Some blood tests are now carried out by the use of reagent strips, for example:

Azostix, which indicates a raised blood urea level.
Dextrostix, a semi-quantitative method for estimating the blood sugar (glucose) levels.

These tests are time-saving, but it is essential that each detail of the instructions is followed. Timing is critical; a watch with a second·hand must be used or the results may be unreliable.

Blood Counts

Blood counts may be made by drawing blood directly from a finger prick into special pipettes which the operator brings to the bedside. More commonly, however, venous blood is collected in a sequestrene tube and two thin blood smears prepared for the differential count in the laboratory. This second method is more convenient, as several other examinations can be made from the same specimen if required. Usually 2–3 ml of blood is collected.

Erythrocyte Sedimentation Rate/Plasma Viscosity Test

The sedimentation rate measures the distance which the red cells fall in one hour when a column of blood is allowed to stand vertically in a glass tube of fine uniform bore. Several different methods are used, and the normal values vary with each method. It is not a diagnostic test, as most infections cause an increase in the rate, but it is very useful in following the course of a disease such as rheumatic fever or tuberculosis. The greater the activity of the disease the higher is the sedimentation rate.

Wintrobe's method is the test most used. 3 ml of blood is placed in a tube containing ammonium and potassium oxalate, and mixed well. The blood is then put into a special Wintrobe sedimentation rate tube and allowed to stand undisturbed for one hour. The height of the column of clear plasma above the sediment of red cells is then measured.

Westergren's method employs a different-sized tube and uses 0–4 ml of 3% sodium citrate solution for the anti-coagulant.

Similar findings can be obtained from the *plasma viscosity test*. This test compares the viscosity of blood with water; in normal blood the viscosity is 20% greater than that of water, in chronic infection and inflammatory diseases the viscosity of blood increases.

Coagulation Blood Tests

The following coagulation tests are used to investigate the possibility of haemorrhagic disease or the effect of anticoagulant drugs.

Platelet count (Normal range: 150 × 10⁹ to 400 × 10⁹/litre) A very low count may occur in acute leukaemia, aplastic anaemia, and thrombocytopenia. The platelet count may increase following surgery, especially splenectomy, which increases the risk of a thrombosis occurring.

Bleeding time The duration of bleeding after puncture of the ear lobe or the anterior aspect of the forearm is between two and five minutes. This time is increased in acute leukaemia and severe pernicious anaemia.

Clotting time   Clotting time is the average time taken for 1 ml of blood to clot in the first three of four test tube samples. The normal clotting time varies between four and seven minutes. It is prolonged in anticoagulant therapy, Christmas disease and obstructive jaundice.

Prothrombin ratio test (prothrombin time)   This test is done on a freshly-collected sample of blood in a citrated tube. Care must be taken to add the right amount of blood and to mix it thoroughly. The ratio in which the result is expressed shows how long it takes for the specimen to coagulate compared with a normal specimen of blood. If it takes twice as long the ratio is 2:1 (this may be stated as a prothrombin *index* of 50%). The desirable ratio for those patients having anticoagulant therapy lies between 9:1 and 3:2. This test is used to monitor anticoagulant therapy.

Bone Marrow Specimen

Samples of bone marrow may be required in cases of pernicious anaemia and leukaemia. These are obtained by an aseptic procedure involving puncturing the manubrium (part of the sternum) or the iliac crest with a sternal puncture needle and aspirating the bone marrow. A member of the laboratory staff comes to the ward with the required equipment. The patient is sedated before the procedure and the nurse remains with the patient throughout.

Plasma Proteins

Disturbances of the plasma proteins occur in many conditions. Abnormally low levels of serum albumin may give rise to oedema and may be the result of liver disease, loss of albumin in the urine in the nephrotic syndrome, or a diet deficient in proteins. Serum protein levels are often low in patients with chronic infections or extensive burns. Raised or abnormal globulins are found in patients with multiple myeloma.

Plasma cortisol estimation

There are eleven known hydroxycorticosteroids in plasma; assessment of plasma cortisol is usually performed in preference to urinary ketosteroids as a specific steroid hormone can then be estimated rather than a complex mixture of steroids and metabolites. This is used as a test of adrenal cortical function in Addison's and Simmond's disease. Levels are usually highest in the morning, so that a suitable time for taking blood, which is collected into a special 10 ml tube, would be between 8 and 9 a.m.

Plasma Electrolytes

See p. 48.

Serous Fluids

Pleural effusions, pericardial effusions and ascites fluid are formed in a number of conditions. Microscopic, bacteriological and chemical investigations of these fluids are used to determine the nature of the underlying disorder.

Cell content In transudates only a small number of cells are present. In pyogenic infection, pus cells are present in large numbers, while in tuberculous infection there is a high percentage of lymphocytes. Red blood cells are often present in malignant disease.

Bacteriological investigation In infective conditions, culture for pyogenic organisms or *Myobacterium tuberculosis* may reveal the organism responsible. For the detection of tuberculous infection the fluids may be injected into guinea-pigs.

Chemical examination The protein content is increased in infective conditions, but may also be raised to a lesser extent in transudates.

Pleural Biopsy

Biopsy of the parietal pleura may be needed in order to determine whether a pleural effusion is tuberculous or malignant in origin. The biopsy needle is usually inserted into the posterior chest wall; the exact site is decided after physical and radiological examination. The patient should sit well forward in the bed with his arms resting on a pillow placed on a bed table in front of him. A labelled specimen jar containing formalin should be available for the biopsy specimen.

Tests of Gastric Function

Tests of gastric function are designed to estimate the hydrochloric acid content of the gastric juice and the amount and content of the gastric residue (resting juice) after a period of fasting. The tests vary from one hospital to another and even according to the doctor who orders them. Some examples are given below.

Diagnex Test (Tubeless Test)

No preparation containing aluminium, calcium, iron or magnesium must be given during the 24 hours prior to the test. The patient should fast for 12 hours before the test begins and should have nothing but the test substances and water by mouth until the test is complete.

1. At a specified time (usually 6 a.m.) the patient is asked to empty the bladder and this urine is discarded.
2. The patient is given capsules containing caffeine sodium benzoate 250 mg with a glass of water; this preparation is a gastric stimulant.
3. If an injection of histamine has been ordered it is given at 6.45 a.m.
4. At 7 a.m. the patient again empties the bladder and the entire amount passed is saved and sent to the laboratory labelled 'control urine'.
5. Immediately after emptying the bladder the patient is given the Diagnex Blue as blue granules suspended in about 60 ml of water. The granules do not dissolve and thus the patient must be instructed not to chew them but to swallow them whole. A further 60 ml of water is given to ensure that no granules are left in the glass.
6. Two hours later, at 9 a.m., the patient empties the bladder and all the urine passed is saved and sent to the laboratory labelled 'test urine'.

If the gastric juice contains hydrochloric acid, an exchange of hydrogen ions occurs between the Diagnex resin and the juice. The resin is then absorbed and excreted in the urine.

The test cannot be repeated until at least a week has elapsed and therefore the nurse should be sure that the instructions are understood and carried out accurately. The patient may continue to pass blue or greenish blue urine for some days after the test.

Pentagastrin Test Meal

The pentagastrin test replaces many of the other former gastric test meals, and is used to estimate the amount of hydrochloric acid secreted by the stomach. The patient is fasted from 9 p.m. the previous evening. Early the following morning a radio-opaque Ryle's tube is passed into the stomach with the usual precautions. The stomach is aspirated every 15 minutes for 1 hour; this aspirate may be discarded. Pentagastrin 6μg/kg body weight is injected subcutaneously using a tuberculin syringe. For the next 1–2 hours the stomach is aspirated every 15 minutes. The volume of the aspirate is recorded, then it is sieved through gauze into a special container provided by the laboratory. On completion of the test all the aspirate collected is sealed in its container, carefully labelled and sent to the laboratory.

Pentagastrin is very similar to the gastric hormone, gastrin, and in normal circumstances stimulates the stomach to produce hydrochloric acid. In cases of peptic ulceration there may be over-secretion of hydrochloric acid; in cases of pernicious anaemia or cancer of the stomach there is likely to be under-secretion (achlorhydria).

Analysis of Faeces

Occult Blood

A small specimen of uncontaminated faeces is sent to
the laboratory in a waxed or plastic container. The
patient should avoid eating red meats for two or three
days prior to the test. False positive results are also
likely if the patient is bleeding slightly from the oral
cavity. The faeces may appear to contain blood
(melaena) as a result of the patient taking iron medication, bismuth or manganese.

In the 'conservative' treatment of gastric or duodenal ulcers it is usual to send repeated specimens until
the result is negative, this being taken to imply that any
upper intestinal bleeding has stopped.

Fat

Specimens of faeces must be inspected before submit-
ting them for quantitive analysis. The highly fluid
stools obtained by means of purgatives and enemas
are useless. No aperients and particularly no oily
preparations such as liquid paraffin should be given
for several days prior to the test. If a barium meal or
enema has been done, all barium must be expelled
from the tract prior to the day of the test. A minimum
uncontaminated specimen of 30 g should be collected
in a waxed container which should be made airtight
before despatch to the laboratory. On a normal diet
the total daily output of fat should be less than 7 g. In
some circumstances estimation of the faecal fat on a
free diet may not provide a sufficiently accurate result
and a fat balance test will be necessary.

Fat balance test   The patient is given a standard diet containing 50 g of fat per day, during the test and for at least 48 hours prior to its commencement. It is essential that all the food is eaten. Any rejects must be weighed and subtracted from the original weight of the diet.

First day: the patient is given two capsules containing carmine before breakfast. The stools are examined as passed and when they are coloured by carmine the whole stool is saved and sent to the laboratory. All subsequent stools for the next six days are saved.

Sixth day: the patient is given 60 g of charcoal powder mixed with water. All stools passed are saved until the charcoal appears in the faeces.

All the specimens are sent to the laboratory for a complete fat balance study. Normally 99% of ingested fat is absorbed. A high fat content in the faeces suggests a malabsorption syndrome, such as coeliac disease.

Other Malabsorption Tests

The absorption of substances other than fat may also be impaired. Carbohydrate absorption is measured by the *xylose tolerance test.* The patient should fast for 12 hours before the test, then take 5 g of xylose (which is a relatively inert carbohydrate) in a drink of fruit juice, after emptying the bladder. All the urine passed in the following five hours is collected and sent to the laboratory. During this time the patient is encouraged to drink water but does not eat. The five-hour specimen of urine should contain at least 1.2 g of xylose. If the uptake of this substance from the gut is impaired, less than this amount will be present in the urine.

A number of vitamins are absorbed from the bowel, and the body may become deficient in them in states of abnormal intestinal function. If vitamin K is absorbed poorly the prothrombin concentration in the plasma falls and a bleeding tendency may develop. Poor absorption of vitamin B12, deficiency of which leads to pernicious anaemia, is tested by administering a very small dose of radioactive vitamin B12 and measuring its excretion in the urine (Schilling test). A similar but much simpler test is the Dicopac test.

Intestinal Biopsy

The intestinal wall is abnormal in conditions such as coeliac disease or idiopathic steatorrhoea. A specimen may be obtained by means of an instrument known as a Crosby capsule. The capsule contains a cutting mechanism controlled through a long thin flexible tube. It is usually swallowed about 10 p.m., the patient having fasted since 6 p.m. From the stomach it progresses about 5 cm per hour. The position is checked in the morning by radiography and the biopsy taken from the appropriate site by applying suction to the tube. The biopsy may also be obtained using a fibreoptic endoscopy instrument, in which case direct visual examination of the site precedes the taking of the biopsy.

Pancreatic Function

The secretion of insulin by the pancreas is disturbed in diabetes mellitus, but is not usually affected by other diseases of the pancreas unless the organ has been extensively destroyed. This aspect of pancreatic function is considered under 'Carbohydrate Metabolism' on p. 197.

The exocrine functions of the pancreas may be tested either by estimating the amylase content of the blood or urine, or by analysis of the duodenal contents for pancreatic enzymes and bicarbonates.

Urinary Amylase

A sample of urine collected over several hours is desirable. However, in an emergency, for example to confirm a diagnosis of acute pancreatitis, examination of the first specimen obtained is permissible. If the urine has to be sent from some distance to the laboratory it should be preserved with benzene. The normal range of urinary amylase is from 6 to 30 units per ml. A value of 200 or more in a case with acute abdominal signs is almost pathognomonic of acute pancreatitis. Intermediate values between 30 and 200, if found regularly, suggest the possibility of pancreatic duct obstruction.

Duodenal Drainage

A more detailed examination of the pancreatic function may be carried out by examination of the juice obtained by duodenal drainage. A weighted duodenal tube is passed into the stomach and a specimen of gastric juice is withdrawn. The patient then lies on his right side to promote the passage of the tube into the duodenum; if necessary the position of the tube can be checked by radiography. When the tube is in the duodenum the contents are aspirated and tested for sodium bicarbonate and the pancreatic enzymes trypsin, amylase and lipase. Pancreatic secretions may be stimulated by an intravenous injection of secretin.

Liver Function Tests

Interpretation of tests of liver function is complex

since the liver has numerous functions, any single one of which may be deficient whilst the others remain relatively intact. Also the liver has a large functional reserve — it has to be very extensively damaged before any of the tests show an abnormal result. No test has yet been devised which tests the liver as a whole, but there are innumerable tests which depend on the different individual functions of the organ; the commonest of these tests are outlined below. (See also 'Serum Enzymes' on p. 201.)

Bile Pigments

Failure of the liver to excrete bile pigments leads to their accumulation in the blood and their excretion in the urine.

Bilirubin

The normal level of bilirubin in the blood serum varies from 5 to 17 μmol/litre. Increased serum bilirubin is found in cases of liver damage, obstructive jaundice and haemolytic jaundice. Bilirubin will be present in the urine in cases of obstructive jaundice.

Urobilinogen This pigment will be present in the urine in cases of incomplete obstructive jaundice, of diffuse liver damage — for example infective hepatitis — and haemolytic jaundice. In cases of complete obstructive jaundice urobilinogen is absent from the urine. For urine tests for bile pigments see p. 167.

Serum Protein Tests

Serum protein tests are designed to show variations from the normal ability of the liver to synthesize serum proteins. They are not specific tests for liver damage since alterations in the serum proteins may be found in many other diseases.

In liver diseases the serum albumin level is low and the serum globulin level is raised. The abnormal composition of the serum proteins is also reflected in the so-called 'empirical liver function tests', for example the thymol turbidity test. These become positive when liver function is impaired, e.g. in cirrhosis of the liver and infective hepatitis.

Bromsulphalein Test

This test measures the ability of the liver to excrete a dye, sulphobromophthalein sodium (Bromsulphalein). The patient should have a fat-free breakfast and no food thereafter until the test is completed. At 10 a.m. 5 mg/kg of body weight of 5% Bromsulphalein is injected intravenously very slowly (over a period of three minutes). The ampoule must be warmed if any crystals are visible. At 10.45 a.m., 10 ml of clotted blood is collected from another vein, special care being taken to avoid haemolysis. After 45 minutes the serum should show that less than 7% of the injected dose is still retained.

Prothrombin Concentration Test

Prothrombin is formed in the liver from vitamin K absorbed from the intestine. A low prothrombin level may be due to liver damage or to the nonabsorption of vitamin K resulting from biliary obstruction. If the prothrombin concentration is low, the test may be repeated after an injection of vitamin K, and if it then returns to normal, biliary obstruction is suspected. (The prothrombin level must also be estimated regularly in patients having anticoagulant therapy.)

Liver Biopsy

Prior to carrying out this investigation the patient's blood group is ascertained, his blood is cross-matched, and the haemoglobin and prothrombin content, the bleeding time and the clotting time are ascertained. The biopsy is not usually performed if the prothrombin content is found to be below 70% of the normal.

The patient lies on his back well over to the right of the bed and a pillow is placed under his left side to tilt the trunk slightly to the right. Bleeding into the peritoneal cavity may occur following liver biopsy and therefore the patient must be kept under close observation. An hourly pulse chart should be kept for at least 12 hours after this procedure.

Renal Function

Ordinary chemical and microscopic examination of the urine, although valuable, gives only limited information as to the condition of the kidneys. Albuminuria, for example, may be due to other than nephritic conditions, and in nephritis it is not always possible to determine from simple chemical examination of the urine whether or not the kidneys are functioning properly. In spite of a large excretion of urea, uric acid, creatinine and other end products of nitrogenous metabolism, the level of these substances in the blood may be above normal. Tests have, therefore, been devised with the object either of directly estimating renal efficiency or of investigating the severity and following the progress of events in renal disease.

Blood Urea Estimation

At least 2.5 ml of blood is collected from a vein into a sequestrene tube to prevent clotting. With smaller quantities of blood reasonable results can be obtained when the urea content is high, but the results in border-line cases cannot be regarded as sufficiently accurate. If this test is done in conjunction with a urinary urea concentration test, the blood sample must be taken before the urea draught is given.

The normal range of blood urea is from 2.5 to 6.6 mmol/litre. Low values occur in normal pregnancy and in acute jaundice, but may also be produced by protein deficiency or by flushing out the system with water as in diabetes insipidus or diuresis produced by high fluid intake. High values nearly always indicate serious renal impairment, but moderate increases can occur due to hydration, circulatory failure and high protein intake without renal involvement. In cases with some degree of renal damage, wide fluctuations in blood urea content can be produced by variations in protein and water intake, so that the fall which occurs when a nephrotic patient is given a low protein diet and a limited fluid intake is not necessarily an indication of fundamental improvement.

Urea Concentration Test (Maclean)

The intake of fluids should be restricted as much as possible from the afternoon preceding the test. No breakfast is allowed.

In the morning, blood is collected for urea estimation (see above) *before* the urea draught is given. The patient empties the bladder and a sample of this urine is placed in a bottle labelled '1'. The patient is then given 15g of urea dissolved in about 60 ml water; a smaller dose is used for children in proportion to age. At intervals of one hour from taking the urea draught the patient empties the bladder. Three specimens (marked '2', '3' and '4') are thus obtained and sent to the laboratory in labelled containers. Specimens sent from a distance should be preserved by adding a few drops of benzene.

Some authorities prefer to discard the urine passed during the first hour after the draught and consider only the results for the second, third and fourth hours. A figure of 2% or over in one or more of the hour specimens is regarded as evidence of satisfactory renal function. Diuresis sometimes prevents this concentration being reached; if the volume exceeds 120 ml a concentration of urea below 2% does not necessarily indicate poor function. The restriction of fluids is designed to prevent diuresis; ignoring the first hour specimen in which diuresis is often most marked, also aims at overcoming this difficulty.

Urea Clearance Test

Two methods are used, one without and one with urea administration, the aim of the latter being to impose a load on the kidneys to provoke maximum efficiency. The need for this is denied by some authorities. In either case the test should be performed before breakfast is taken. The details of these tests may vary in different hospitals. Two methods are given below.

First method (without urea administration)

8 a.m.   The patient empties the bladder completely. Discard the urine.

9 a.m.   The patient empties the bladder completely. Place the *whole* specimen directly, without

measurement, into a container. Mark the bottle 'A'.

A specimen of blood is collected immediately for urea estimation.

10 a.m. The patient again empties the bladder completely. Place the *whole* specimen directly, without measurement, into a container. Mark the bottle 'B'.

Second method (with urea administration)

8 a.m. The patient empties the bladder. Discard the urine. Give immediately a draught containing 15 g of urea (a smaller dose for children according to age).

9 a.m. The patient empties the bladder completely. Discard this urine.

9.45 a.m. A specimen of blood is collected for urea estimation.

10 a.m. The patient empties the bladder completely. Place the *whole* specimen directly, without measurement, into a clean bottle.

Greater sensitivity is claimed for this second test, but, as might be expected, this increased sensitivity will not be realized in practice unless close attention is given to detail.

The patient must be asked to make special efforts to empty the bladder completely at the times specified. These times must be noted accurately — to the nearest minute — and recorded on the slip to accompany the specimens to the laboratory. The intervals need not be precisely one hour if this is done. The urine must be poured as carefully as possible into the specimen bottles, for the total amount is accurately measured in the laboratory and any loss of urine will produce a low result. The specimens of urine may be preserved if necessary by the addition of three or four drops of benzene. In the case of children and unusually small or large adults the height and weight may also be required by the laboratory for the calculation of the result.

Analysis of the specimens submitted gives figures from which the efficiency of the kidneys is calculated, the result being in terms of the percentage of average normal renal function. The common range in normal health is from 75 to 120%.

Cases of acute nephritis have been studied by means of this test. The patients show a marked fall in the urea clearance, sometimes as low as 10% during the early weeks of the acute stage and, while fatal cases show a continued fall, a rise in the clearance value is accompanied by clinical improvement. The active chronic phase of the disease is indicated by a progressively diminishing urea clearance, uraemia and death being imminent when values below 10% are obtained. The renal failure found in some cases of hypertension is also associated with a falling urea clearance, while in nephrosis no impairment of function is found.

With this, as with all other tests of kidney function, the result indicates the state of affairs on the day of the test only, although the condition may be changing extremely rapidly.

Urine Concentration Test

No fluids are allowed from 4 p.m. on the preceding day until 8 a.m. on the morning of the test. The patient empties his bladder at 8, 9 and 10 a.m. and the volume and specific gravity of each specimen is measured. The specific gravity of at least one specimen should exceed 1.025 if renal function is normal. This test should not be done if the blood urea is raised.

Renal Biopsy

Prior to this procedure an X-ray examination is carried out in order to obtain information about the size and position of the kidneys, the patient's blood group is ascertained, his blood is cross-matched and the haemoglobin content estimated.

The patient lies in the prone position with a sandbag under the abdomen to fix the kidney against the dorsal surface of the body.

The site of the biopsy is usually the lower pole of the right kidney and its position is ascertained by a fine exploring needle inserted after the injection of a local anaesthetic.

Haematuria is not uncommon after renal biopsy; the appearance of blood in the urine, even if slight in amount, should be reported at once. An hourly pulse chart should be kept for at least 12 hours.

Other Investigations Performed on Urine

Ascorbic Acid Saturation Test

This is carried out on patients with ascorbic acid deficiency, who may take more than seven days to reach saturation. It is repeated daily until the patient excretes more than 30 mg of ascorbic acid in the two-hour specimen.

8 a.m.	The patient empties the bladder and is given 700 mg ascorbic acid by mouth.
12 noon	The patient empties the bladder and the specimen is discarded.

2 p.m.   The patient empties the bladder and all the
            urine passed is collected into a special con-
            tainer (which contains 50 ml of glacial acetic
            acid). The ascorbic acid content must be
            estimated within one hour.

Figlu Test

This is carried out to detect folic acid deficiency.
Histadine monohydrochloride 15 g is given by mouth
after overnight fasting and food is withheld until one
hour after administration of the dose. As histadine is
only slightly soluble it is administered by mixing it
with water until all has been taken. Three hours after
taking the dose, the patient voids urine and this is
discarded. All urine passed over the next five hours
(i.e. from three to eight hours after the histadine dose)
is collected into a special container which contains
N/10 hydrochloric acid and a few crystals of thymol.

Catecholamines

To estimate the amines, adrenaline and noradrenaline
in the urine in suspected cases of phaeochromocyto-
ma (a tumour of the adrenal medulla), a 24-hour
specimen of urine is collected in a special container in
which there is dilute acid.

17-Ketosteroids (Oxosteroids) and 17-Ketogenic Steroids (Oxogenic Steroids)

These are tests of adrenal cortical dysfunction which
are carried out on a 24-hour specimen collection of
urine.

Bence Jones Protein

This test is used in the diagnosis of multiple myeloma and secondary cancer of bone. A 24-hour specimen of urine is required from the patient; it is concentrated to 300 times and tested by a special anti-serum. This test may show the presence of abnormal proteins in the urine before changes appear in the bone marrow.

Slide Pregnancy Test

Early morning urine is best for this test as it is more concentrated. It should be collected in a sterile bottle and sent to the laboratory without delay. Some laboratories accept a bottle which has previously been boiled and is free from detergent. The test is not normally positive until approximately 41 days from the date of the last menstrual period.

Cerebrospinal Fluid

For complete routine examination 5–10 ml of cerebrospinal fluid should be sent to the laboratory. Points to be borne in mind in collecting these specimens include:

1. Contamination with blood detracts from the value of the report in proportion to the amount present.
2. Dilution of the cerebrospinal fluid with water, saline, spirit and other fluids must be rigorously avoided.
3. Bacterial contamination invalidates some of the tests, such as the sugar content test and the colloidal gold test.

Cell count In normal fluid there are usually a few white cells (lymphocytes) present, up to 5000/ml. Pus

cells are found in pyogenic infections, and lymphocytes are increased in tuberculous meningitis, syphilitic infections and poliomyelitis. Red blood cells will be
found in cases of subarachnoid haemorrhage, and in
cerebral haemorrhage if blood has leaked into the
ventricles.

Protein   The concentration of protein is increased in
infective conditions, syphilitic lesions and spinal block.

Glucose   The normal range is from 3.3 to 4.4 mmol/
litre. Glucose is usually low or absent in infective and
tuberculous meningitis. Slightly raised values are said
to occur in encephalitis lethargica. The spinal fluid
sugar is also raised in subjects with raised blood
sugar.

Sodium chloride   The normal range is from 120 to
130 mmol/litre. Values tend to be reduced in acute
meningitis and in the late stages of tuberculous
meningitis. In syphilitic conditions normal values are
common.

Lange's colloidal gold reaction   No precipitation of
gold occurs with normal fluid in any dilution. The
degree of precipitation, when it occurs, is reported
numerically, 0 indicating no precipitation and 5 complete precipitation. In general paralysis of the insane
the gold is precipitated by the lower dilutions in a
standard series, the results report being of the type 5 5
5 5 4 2 1 0 0 0 0 (paretic curve), while meningitic fluids
usually show the greatest change in the higher dilutions, the report reading 0 0 0 0 2 3 5 5 5 5 5.

Carbohydrate Metabolism

The following tests are used to detect disturbances of carbohydrate metabolism, in particular diabetes mellitus.

Estimation of Blood Sugar

Blood sugar tests should be done in the morning before food has been taken. If the patient is unable to visit the laboratory, 0.5 ml of blood may be sent to the laboratory in a special container containing a preservative mixture. The tube is thoroughly shaken to ensure the blood mixes with the preservative, since the sugar content in the blood begins to diminish within one hour. Where repeated observations are to be made, as during adjustment of insulin or diet, specimens must always be collected in the same relation to the previous meal and insulin injection, in order that the results may be comparable. This may be either three hours after a meal, or in the morning before breakfast.

The great majority of normal fasting blood sugar values lie between 2.5 and 4.7 mmol/litre. It has been found that, almost without exception, values of 7.2 mmol/litre or more are found only in those cases which give a 'diabetic curve' in the glucose tolerance test (see below). Some cases of hyperthyroidism, or patients taking thyroxine also give high results, whilst apprehension over appearing at the laboratory for the first time is occasionally responsible. Very low values are found after an excessive dose of insulin, following severe exercise, or in the rare condition of hyperinsulinism.

Glucose Tolerance Test

The way in which the individual is able to deal with a standard quantity of sugar affords valuable information as to the presence or otherwise of a diabetic tendency. It is desirable that the test should be done in the morning before food has been taken, and extremes of high or low carbohydrate intake should be avoided for at least one day before the test. Nervous tension and rush before and during the test should be discouraged and smoking must be forbidden.

The patient may be sent to the laboratory by appointment for the test. Where this is not practicable the following procedure must be adopted:

1. The patient empties the bladder. A sample of this urine is placed in a bottle marked 'A'.
2. A 0.5 ml sample of blood is collected in a special blood sugar tube (see previous section).
3. 50 g of glucose is given dissolved in 100 ml of water (for children, the amount of glucose is related to their weight).
4. At half hour intervals thereafter, five more samples of blood are collected.
5. The patient empties the bladder one hour and two hours after the administration of glucose; these specimens are labelled 'B' and 'C'.

When the urine specimens are sent some distance to the laboratory for testing they should be preserved with a few drops of benzene. A normal individual should show a fasting sugar level of between 2.5 and 4.7 mmol/litre, a definite rise during the first hour and a return to fasting limits within two hours. The maximum reading should not exceed 9 mmol/litre and no sugar should be found in the specimens of urine. In the various uncommon conditions in which reducing substances other than glucose are present in the urine, for example pentose, the tolerance test usually gives a normal result.

Diabetes mellitus   The blood sugar level may initially be normal or raised. After the administration of glucose it will rise to a sustained level of about 9 mmol/litre, and remain above the fasting range for more than two hours. In the majority of diabetic patients, the first specimen of urine, A, contains no sugar, but sugar appears in the later specimens B and C.

Renal glycosuria   In this condition, the initial blood sugar level is normal or subnormal. It does not rise above 9 mmol/litre and the return to fasting limits is not delayed, being often more rapid than usual. Sugar is not present in the first specimen of urine except in unusual cases with very low renal threshold, but is invariably present in the second specimen. It is almost universally agreed that this fairly common condition is of no pathological significance. One of the values of the glucose tolerance test lies in recognizing these cases and saving them the rigours of diabetic treatment.

Hyperthyroid and pituitary disturbances   Abnormal blood sugar curves are sometimes found in these conditions.

Glycosuria of pregnancy   In a fair percentage of normal pregnancies glycosuria is found while the blood sugar remains normal.

Calcium Metabolism

The causes of disturbed calcium metabolism include diseases of the parathyroid glands, failure of absorption of calcium due to steatorrhoea, vitamin D deficiency and chronic renal disease.

In the condition of hyperparathyroidism due to tumours of the parathyroid glands, calcium is lost from the bones, leading to osteomalacia and a raised serum calcium level. In these cases, the blood phosphorus is low and the alkaline phosphatase level in the blood is raised. In hypoparathyroidism blood calcium is low, which may lead to tetany. In steatorrhoea there is a failure of absorption of calcium from the gut which gives rise to low blood calcium and osteomalacia. The administration of vitamin D aids calcium absorption, but excessive dosage can cause a raised level of calcium in the blood.

Laboratory tests used in disordered calcium metabolism include estimation of the blood calcium, the blood phosphorus, the blood alkaline phosphatase, and the calcium balance. This last test involves a somewhat complicated routine as described below.

Calcium Balance Collection

This test consists of collecting separate specimens of urine and faeces over a period of three or four days. Prior to the collection of these specimens there is an 'equilibrium period' of four to six days.

During the equilibrium period the patient is prescribed a weighed and balanced diet which is strictly monitored by the dietician. The choice of food is very limited, all the food offered must be eaten, and nothing extra is permitted once the diet is commenced. The food is cooked in distilled water in utensils reserved for this purpose. There is no limit to the amount of water the patient may drink but it must be distilled, and distilled mouthwashes should replace toothpaste. Substances which may artificially raise the urinary or faecal calcium levels are excluded. Prescribed medication should also be considered for its calcium content and advice sought on the administration of any medication during the collection period, particularly aperients. This equilibrium period may last from four to six days and during this time minor adjustments may be made to the diet.

The evening prior to the collection of the first specimen, a carmine dye is taken orally which colours the faeces red.

On the first day of collection, the patient empties the bladder on waking and this specimen of urine is discarded. All other urine passed in the next 24 hours is collected into a single container provided by the pathology department. One or more of these specimens may be required.

Similarly the faeces are collected over a 24-hour period. A separate container is required for each 24-hour period. Collection of faeces is made easier by lining the bedpan with cellophane. The specimen must not be contaminated by urine, and the patient should be counselled and assisted whenever necessary. Oral carmine dye is administered after the second and fourth specimens have been collected.

Calcium estimation of both urinary and faecal specimens are compared to the dietary calcium intake to see if the patient has achieved a balance between intake and output. (See Normal values, p. 207.)

This routine may be modified to allow balance tests of other substances such as faecal fat to be carried out.

Serum Enzymes

A vast number of enzymes are involved in cellular processes, but only very small amounts are found in the blood. When cells, particularly those in muscle and liver, are damaged, however, the concentration of certain enzymes in the blood rises and estimation of the relevant enzyme helps to establish the existence or amount of cellular damage. Two of the most commonly estimated are aspartate transaminase (AST — also known as serum glutamic oxaloacetic transaminase or SGOT), which is increased especially after myocardial infection and in hepatitis, and alanine transaminase (ALT — also known as serum glutamic pyruvic transaminase or SGPT), which is increased in various forms of liver cell damage.

Phosphatase

Two forms of phosphatase enzyme are present in blood serum, the alkaline and the acid form. The former is increased in bone diseases, such as hyper-parathyroidism, bone tumours and Paget's disease; the latter is frequently increased in carcinoma of the prostate gland with secondary deposits. The laboratory should be told which form is to be investigated when sending the specimen.

Either form of phosphatase can be determined on the serum obtained from 5–6 ml of blood. The normal ranges vary with the method used for determination and therefore this information will be provided by the laboratory.

Thyroid Function Tests

The function of the thyroid gland can be assessed by measuring the level of thyroxine in the blood. Also of value is the level of protein-bound iodine (PBI) in the blood, which is normally 4–7.5 μg/dl.

Radioactive Iodine

The size of the thyroid and the distribution of activity within it can be determined using radioactive iodine. A measured tracer dose of radioactive iodine (^{131}I) is given orally or occasionally intravenously, and the amount of 'take up' or concentration of the radioactive material by the thyroid gland is recorded by a Geiger counter sited over the thyroid area two hours later. A patient with myxoedema is asked to return 24 hours after the administration of the radioactive iodine, as the 'take up' is much slower.

The results of the test may be invalidated if the patient is given radiological contrast media, food containing iodine, thyroid preparations, perchlorates or thiocyanates, or radioactive isotopes. Some of these preparations may affect the result of the test even if a considerable time elapses between their discontinuation and the test, for example Lugol's iodine and contrast media; it is therefore advisable to have a clear interval of four weeks if possible before carrying out the test.

The patient should be given the following instructions:

1. No food containing iodine, such as onions, watercress or fish, should be eaten for at least two days before coming for the test.
2. Iodized throat tablets, cough linctus and any proprietary food with a high iodine content should also be avoided. If these have been taken during the past month, the department should be informed at the time of making the appointment.
3. A light breakfast may be taken on the morning of the test.

Thyroglobulin Antibody (T.A.) Test

Thyroglobulin antibody in the serum is associated with certain forms of hypothyroidism; primary myxoedema and Hashimoto's disease. The test requires 2 ml of clotted blood.

24
Normal Biochemical Values in Adults

Blood Plasma or Serum

For electrolytes see p. 48.

Test	Normal Value
Alkali reserve (HCO_3)	21–32 mmol/litre
Bilirubin (Indirect van den Bergh)	5–17 µmol/litre
Calcium	2.12–2.62 mmol/litre
Cholesterol	3.6–7.8 mmol/litre
Chloride	95–105 mmol/litre
Creatinine	62–124 µmol/litre

Enzymes and transaminases

Acid phosphatase total	less than 8.2 IU/litre (International Units)
prostatic	less than 7.2 IU/litre (King Armstrong units)
Alkaline phosphatase	8–27 IU/litre (Bodansky units)
Alanine transaminase (SGPT)	5–30 IU/litre (Reitman-Frankel units)
Aspartate transaminase (SGOT)	5–30 IU/litre (Reitman-Frankel units)
Creatine kinase (CPK)	less than 130 IU/litre
2-Hydroxybutyrate dehydrogenase (HBD)	150–325 IU/litre
Lactate dehydrogenase (LDH)	240–525 IU/litre (McQueen units)
Non-protein nitrogen	14–21 mmol/litre

Protein

Albumin	36–52 g/litre
Globulin	24–37 g/litre

Fibrinogen	1.5–4 g/litre
Total protein (whole blood)	62–82 g/litre
Specific gravity	1.023–1.028 (36–43 nmol/litre)
Urea	2.5–6.6 mmol/litre
Uric acid	0.15–0.45 mmol/litre

Blood Count

Test	Normal Value
Haemoglobin	13.5–18 g/dl (men)
	11.5–16.4 g/dl (women)
Platelets	150×10^9–400×10^9/litre
Red cell count	4.5×10^{12}–6×10^{12}/litre (men)
	3.9×10^{12}–5.6×10^{12}/litre (women)
White cell count	4×10^9–11×10^9/litre

Cerebrospinal Fluid (CSF)

Test	Normal Value
Pressure	80–180 mm of water
Volume	120–140 ml
Chloride	120–130 mmol/litre
Glucose	3.3–4.4 mmol/litre
Protein	0.15–0.40 g/litre

Faeces

Test	Normal Value
Estimated daily weight	60–250 g
Dry weight	20–60 g

Nitrogen	71–143 mmol/24 hours
Fat	
total	10–27%
split	11–18 mmol/24 hours
neutral	1–6 mmol/24 hours
Porphyrins	0.9–8.8 μmol/24 hours
Trypsin	0–2000 units/4 hours
Urobilinogen	
(stercobilinogen)	50–504 μmol/24 hours

Urine

Test	Normal Value
Amylase (diastase)	80–2000 IU/24 hours
Calcium	2.5–7.5 mmol/24 hours
Chloride	150–170 mmol/litre
Creatine	0–400 μmol/24 hours
Creatinine	9–17 mmol/24 hours
pH	very variable (4.7–8.0)
Phosphate	30–90 mmol/litre
Potassium	35–90 mmol/litre
Sodium	110–240 mmol/litre
Specific gravity	1.000–1.030 (ward testing with urinometer)
Urea	250–600 mmol/24 hours
Volume	600–2000 ml/24 hours

Index

suicide? despair?

who cares?

TELEPHONES COUNTRYWIDE
ARE MANNED—
DAY AND NIGHT—BY

the samaritans

Are you ordinary enough to be one of them?

You need to be a good listener, who understands how other people feel and wants to help them as a friend.

If you are found suitable you will be given the necessary preparation and supervision.

If you feel you might not be able to cope but would like to try, you are probably the type we are looking for.

The Samaritans, too, need friends. To support what they do you can collect or subscribe money and do other administrative duties which they have not time to carry out themselves.

SEE YOUR
TELEPHONE DIRECTORY
FOR CONTACT

And REMEMBER, if you are suicidal or despairing, you can talk to the Samaritans in complete confidence, any hour—day or night.

GL.202

Also available from Baillière Tindall/W.B. Saunders

Medical-Surgical Nursing and Related Physiology (2/e)
J.E. Watson

Both theory and practice are well integrated in this comprehensive second edition. The book emphasizes physiologic concepts as a basis for practising medical and surgical nursing. In addition to an updated chapter on shock, there is coverage of patients' rights, response to illness, physical assessment and monitoring, immunological response, cancer and unconsciousness.

Contents: Patient-Centred Care—Rehabilitation of the Disabled—Causes and Effects of Disease—Infection—Fluid and Electrolyte Balance; Acid-Base Balance—Body Temperature—The Patient with Pain—The Patient with Cancer—The Unconscious Patient—Preoperative and Postoperative Nursing—Age: Implications for Nursing—Nursing in Blood Dycrasias—Nursing in Cardiovascular Disease—Shock—Respiratory Disorders—Disorders of the Alimentary Canal—Disorders of the Liver and Biliary Tract—Disorders of the Pancreas—Disorders of the Urinary System—Disorders of the Reproductive System—Disorders of the Breast—Disorders of the Endocrine System—Disorders of the Nervous System—Bone Disorders—Joint and Collagen Disease—Skin Disorders and Burns—Disorders of the Eye—Disorders of the Ear

W.B. Saunders
0 7216 9136 6   HB   1042pp   116 ills   1979

Baillière's Midwives' Dictionary (7/e)
M. Adams

This well-known pocket reference book provides invaluable source material for midwives and students of midwifery, basic neonatal intensive care and gynaecology. The new edition features:

- new techniques
- neonatal intensive care
- drugs
- many new illustrations
- the U.K.C.C.
- the normal baby
- S.I. Units
- immunization
- new syllabus of training in the UK
- reorganization of the N.H.S.

Baillière Tindall
0 7020 0931 8   PB   368pp   83 ills   1983

Mayes' Midwifery (10/e)
B.R. Sweet

This book for students and trained midwives is a completely revised text incorporating new illustrations. The tenth edition is much more patient centred than previous editions, reflecting the current approach to care of the individual mother and her family.

Baillière Tindall
0 7020 0919 9   PB   630pp   197 ills   1982

Anaesthesia in Midwifery
R. Bevis

Written primarily for the midwife this book supplies much needed information on obstetric anaesthesia, including epidural block. There is also an interesting section devoted to infant resuscitation—a subject of interest to all midwives.

Baillière Tindall
0 7020 1023 5   PB   171pp   29 ills   1983